THE CELLULITE SOLUTION

A Wholistic Guide for a Beautiful Body

Laura Simms

Natural Press
San Clemente
California

THE CELLULITE SOLUTION

A Wholistic Guide for a Beautiful Body

Front cover and illustrations by Joan Soderlund

Editor: Wilhelmine Hartnack

Exerpt on page 118 is from <u>You Can Heal Your Life</u>,
by Lousie L. Hay, © 1984,
Hay House, Inc., Santa Monica, CA
Used by permission.

Library of Congress Catalog Card Number:
91-067052

ISBN 0-9625499-0-8

Printed in the United States
by Delta Lithograph Co.

Natural Press
638 Camino de los Mares, C-240
San Clemente, CA 92673

i

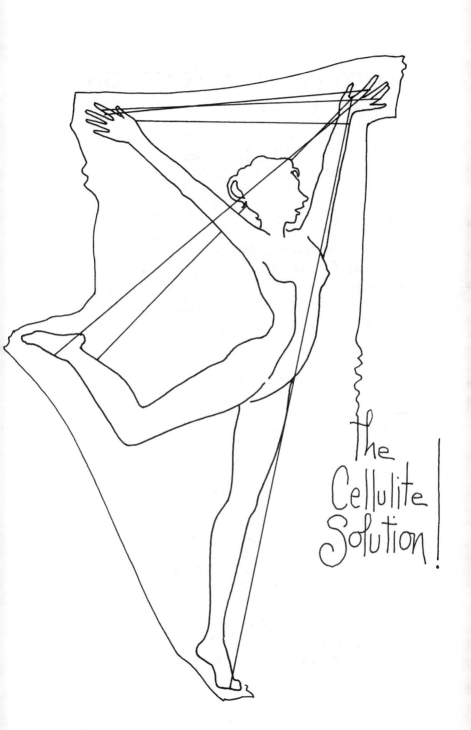

the
Cellulite
Solution!

DISCLAIMER

This book covers certain procedures, treatments, as well as health and beauty products which may be beneficial to some individuals, but contraindicated for others.

Before starting any diet or exercise program, or type of treatment, please consult with your physician regarding your specific needs.

This book is dedicated to my family,
to those of you committed to growth
in your personal lives,
and especially to my husband Ken.

ACKNOWLEDGEMENTS

Thank you, Ara Norwood, for your continuous guidance, encouragement and valuable friendship.

Thank you, Dr. Holly Gahn, Dr. Robert Gahn, E.J.McVay, Vicki Stern, Cassandra Holmes, Dolly Orme-Johnson, Barbara Perry, Nancy Wing, Bob Cassella, Lee Bessa, Gretchen Simms and Jeff Lassek for all of your help, advice and enthusiasm.

Thank you, Omi. Without your knowledge and interest in health this book might never have been inspired.

Thank you, Joe Weider, for introducing the principles of strength training to women through your magazines and books.

Thank you, Joan Soderlund, for your fantastic artwork and illustrations.

Thank you Ken and Mom, for your incredible support, help and encouragement.

Thank you to The Natural Grocer, The Center for Health and Well Being, and other outfits making beneficial contributions to their community.

And especially, thanks to my family, who has loved and supported me all the way.

THE CELLULITE SOLUTION

A Wholistic Guide for a Beautiful Body

Laura Simms

TABLE OF CONTENTS

FOREWORD
DR. HOLLY GAHN

The Cellulite Solution is the most comprehensive book on cellulite ever written. The writer draws from a wealth of personal experiences that enable her to relate to the drama and feelings other women with cellulite experience on a level that is unparalleled. In addition, the information in The Cellulite Solution has been well researched, the data well documented, and put into an easy-to-follow format that enables the lay person as well as the professional to obtain full benefit.

The information contained in this book is both *Holistic* (connoting "natural") and *Wholistic* (meaning taking a "whole body" approach). As a wholistic and holistic practitioner myself, I realize the importance in taking these two approaches. For any program to be effective, whether healing a disease or preventing one, as many of the variables involved as possible must be taken into consideration. Our bodies have spiritual, mental, energetic, structural and chemical aspects. Prof. Worsley, a noted authority on Oriental Medicine in England, compares our body to an orchestra: Each section has a particular function. If one section is out of balance, or out of tune, the other sections are affected adversely too. They must all play together harmoniously.

When a physician treats only one aspect of the disharmony, s/he may get results, but they are generally not as strong or long-lasting. For example: A woman comes into the office complaining of upper back, shoulder and neck pain. The structure of her spine is found to be misaligned. Through Chiropractic manipulation, the bones are put back into place. But this may not have been the full story. Most likely there are emotional factors involved. Many people store their stress in their shoulders. People often store anger or frustration there too. So the emotional aspects must also be explored. Is this woman nourishing the muscles that support her spinal alignment by good nutrition, or are there chemical deficiencies aggravating her condition? What kind of toxic build-ups (like lactic acid crystallizations) are involved, which would inhibit full recovery?

Every possible variable must be considered for total well-being and recovery. This example includes only a few of the aspects that a holistic physician must explore to achieve these results, but if the other variables are addressed at the same time, cure is achieved quicker and is longer lasting.

The closer to nature we are, the less we encounter side effects with anything we do. Likewise, the further we deviate from the way God intended us to use things, the more we can expect bad side effects - toxic reactions, disease, frustration, etc. A Holistic practitioner uses remedies, exercises and other healing practices designed to work with the body the way nature intended.

The Cellulite Solution takes both a Holistic viewpoint by incorporating natural solutions to cellulite, as well as a Wholistic viewpoint by incorporating many of the other variables involved. If the reader truly wants the best and quickest results, she will use as many variables as possible.

Having many of these approaches addressed also gives the reader choices. These choices make it easier to maintain a somewhat 'normal' lifestyle without feeling like she is sacrificing 'everything'. The reader can choose to do as many or as few of the exercises, supplementation, cleansing programs, etc. as she feels comfortable doing. We like choices. The Cellulite Solution gives plenty.

A few years ago when I had a cellulite problem and sought help, there seemed to be only one solution: I went to a spa. There they put me on a rolling drum with 'bumps' on it. The drum pounded and pounded at my legs. I did this for several weeks combined with aerobics with no results. I decided then that there had to be more to cellulite than was given credit. I was right. The Cellulite Solution is a refreshing answer to all my questions and an end to my frustrations with this ego-deflating dis-ease!

Disease is simply a state of dis-ease. It is the body's warning signal that the body is out of balance. Cellulite is a dis-ease. This subject is well addressed in the Cellulite Solution by an author who's conviction and determination to cure herself as well as to help thousands of women, make this book the best of its type on the market!

Holly A. Gahn, O.M.D., L.Ac., Dip.Ac. (NACCA), M.H.

Center for Health and Well Being
Mission Viejo, CA

February 19,1990

PREFACE

"Can you *ever* get rid of cellulite?" Surprised by the voice that seemed to be directed at me, I looked up from my Lifecycle at the frustrated face of a young woman. I was sitting there cycling, reading my book, and along came a woman I had never met to ask me a most *personal* question.

"Well, yes, " I answered, still not quite sure that I was the person she meant to address. "In fact, I once wondered the same thing. Then I discovered that there is most definitely something that can be done about it. It's no big secret, it's only that no one has written a book about it ... yet..." We then began a lengthy and encouraging discussion on the topic of cellulite. We talked about how it develops, about all the solutions and quick fix hypes that are available, as well as the importance of diet and exercise. When we were through talking, I noticed that I had completed twice the time on my Lifecycle that I had intended!

That incident occurred shortly after I had begun to ponder the possibility of putting into print what I had personally learned about cellulite. Since several friends had also questioned me about it, I decided that the Universe was nudging me to get this information out. I knew it was time to stop thinking about it so much, and write about it instead.

In this book you will find a whole-body/mind approach that can help you release cellulite forever. It is both informational and practical. Not only will you find researched information on cellulite, but you will also find helpful exercises, dietary guidelines and techniques. I've attempted to leave no stone unturned; however, should you have any questions, please feel free to write me, in care of the publisher.

Chapter 1

YES, YOU CAN
GET RID OF CELLULITE

Very little information is available on the topic of cellulite. Few people recognize it for what it is, what causes it, and most importantly, how to eliminate it.

Most women believe that once this disfiguring substance develops under their skin, they are stuck with it for life. They consider it to be a part of aging, yet photos of the natives of Polynesian or African cultures never show cellulite. After reading this material, you will realize that you can get rid of cellulite!

A minimum of three weeks as a total commitment is necessary for success in this program. At that point you should already have noticeable results. You should also have developed the habits that will see you through the program until your cellulite is completely gone. Skimming through the entire manual

1

before beginning the program will give you a feel for the kind of diet, exercise, and self-care changes you will be making.

If the information seems overwhelming to you, just remember to take it one step at a time. **The most powerful thing you can do is to begin the <u>strength-training</u> portion of the Anti-Cellulite Exercise Program.**

Keep reminding yourself of how good you feel during the course of the program. **The Cellulite Solution is NOT about self-deprivation; it is about self-nurturing**. Too many women get trapped into the notion that a healthy change is a difficult and punishing one. This is not true about the Anti-Cellulite Program. This program is about rewarding yourself with the best body you could possibly have!

The reason for this book is YOU. I have found the answer for myself. However, I know too many women who are plagued on a daily basis by the ugly, lumpy substance that distracts from their natural, beautiful shape. They too should have access to a solution. Here it is.

Use this book as a reference guide, always available to answer questions as they come up. You will notice that as you master certain sections of the manual, you will be drawn to new information that you may not have noticed during a previous reading.

ATTENTION: WOMEN!

This book is for women. It's for all kinds of women...not just the ones who want a magazine model's body. Some heavier women like their shape and want to keep it (only without the cellulite). Getting rid of the cellulite for them would mean smoothing out the fat and releasing the lumps and bumps. It is, however, more difficult to eliminate cellulite with higher body-fat levels. For women who are already thin, this program means reclaiming their linear, uninterrupted figure.

The Cellulite Solution is for fat women, thin women, black, red, white and yellow women, tall women and short women. *It's for you.* It's not to please men, or the world, or anyone else. Just you.

Cellulite is not merely a question of vanity, it is a question of health. But eliminating it may begin with a concern for one's personal appearance. If you want to change for good, it must be an act of self-love, not self-loathing or disgust. You can start by loving and accepting yourself as you are right now.

ATTENTION: MEN!

To any man who may be reading this, The Cellulite Solution has been written primarily for women. However, a few men do

3

have cellulite, and the information here may benefit you as well. If you do not have cellulite and you are reading this book, you may develop a better understanding and compassion for the struggle that women often have with cellulite and body-image.

This is also your opportunity to support and encourage your female partners. Even though you may not have cellulite, following the principles can be both beneficial and healthy for you, too.

THIN WOMEN HAVE CELLULITE TOO

Heavy women are not the only ones with cellulite. Most women, both fat and thin, have been plagued with at least some cellulite. How many of you have had an aerobics instructor who seemed to be in good shape, until you noticed when she began jumping and bouncing on the exercise floor, the cellulite on the back of her legs jiggled and shook right along with her?

Eighty per cent of adult women have cellulite. Because of this, most women have also accepted cellulite as a normal part of a woman's body. But it is not normal. It's a suggestion that something is out of balance. We need to find out what that is and do something about it.

A WHOLISTIC APPROACH

I want to stress that every application of this program is vitally important, and for the most dramatic results you will do well to follow the instructions in each section exactly. Following only one specific guideline, for example the Anti-Cellulite Diet, will provide you with only partial results. If you want to be completely and permanently free of cellulite, the best approach is the whole body/mind approach presented in The Cellulite Solution.

MY STORY

I first noticed cellulite on my body at the age of twenty. I was about fifteen pounds over my ideal weight, but most disturbing to me were the lumps, bumps and ripples all over my otherwise healthy body. How could it be? I thought this only happened to *older ladies*. I was also convinced that this cellulite would only increase with age. I cringed, imagining my body as it might look in a swimsuit ten years hence, certain that I would need to restrict my summer attire to full body coverage.

The one thing I knew I *could* do was to lose some weight. So I put myself on a restricted 600 calorie per day diet. I also began doing light aerobic exercise such as walking and swimming. After two weeks of much effort and starvation, I weighed myself again. I had barely lost one pound! This was extremely frustrating. I thought my metabolism might have dropped from much of my dieting over the last seven years, but this was ridiculous!

Just as I was ready to give up, a friend persuaded me to join a local gym with her. I began to use Lifecycles, exercise machines, and the free weight equipment for at least an hour a day, six days a week.

Although I had always done my best to avoid intense physical exercise in the past, this was different. There was no competition, no required rate at which to proceed, and the feeling was actually exhilarating.

My metabolism began to pick up and my weight began to drop. I felt a new sense of mental clarity and enthusiasm for life. Could it be? Was the cellulite on my body also diminishing?! It certainly appeared to be.

During this time I also purchased some magazines that changed my life. Joe Weider's *Muscle and Fitness* and *Shape* Magazines were invaluable resources in learning to reshape and redesign my own body. These fitness magazines showed photographs of women with the most amazing bodies I had ever seen. They were lean, healthy, and most incredible of all, not one of these women showed a trace of cellulite.

I wanted to look like them. My desire to look as good as these women grew as I began to read about their lifestyles. I studied their exercise schedules, diets, as well as their food supplement usage. I began to do exactly as they had done.

Upon reading magazine after magazine, and also many books, I began to notice patterns. A consistent thread ran through the lifestyles of these women. It was a matter of inner conviction. Many of these women discovered strength training as a result of feeling frustrated with their overweight, cellulite ridden bodies. As they applied the components of a fitness lifestyle, they developed a commitment to their exercise programs, specialized diets, and especially to their thoughts and attitudes about themselves.

In just three months of copying these patterns, my weight dropped from 136 to 120 pounds, but even better, I had no more cellulite. I felt better than I ever had in my life.

I am not naturally thin and cellulite-free. I began with a problem as bad as most of you reading this, and I refused to accept it for life. If you are a willing to make some lifestyle changes that will keep you healthy and free of cellulite, you have everything you will ever need in your hands right now. Should you give up the program at any point, the cellulite will gradually return, just as surely as it will disappear once you begin practicing the principles again.

THE PROBLEMS

I believe that cellulite is a symptom indicating certain imbalances in the body. The first of these is an overabundance of fat and refined foods in the diet. The second is the possibility of a metabolic disorder, and therefore the body's inability to properly metabolize fats and calories. The third is a congested lymphatic system, which is primarily responsible for keeping the body free of toxic build-up.

Other imbalances are due to genetic factors, fluid retention, poor circulation as well as weak connective tissue. As we explore these, we will discover one very important fact which is receiving increasing attention of the medical profession. **Most of these imbalances stem from an excess of free radicals (toxins) in the body**. The next chapter will discuss how this happens and how it affects the body's state of balance.

THE PLAN

* You will eat a cleansing diet, free of fatty, refined foods and drinks. Instead you will eat foods high in nutrients and fiber.

* You will work to improve the metabolic process through the use of proper diet, exercise, supplements and creative visualization.

* Your body and especially your lymphatic system will be properly cleared of excess toxins and blockages, through the implementation of special techniques, inner cleansing and exercise.

THIS PROGRAM WORKS!

Chapter 2

THE MULTIPLE CAUSES
OF CELLULITE

CELLULITE DOESN'T EXIST!
(I beg your pardon?)

"There's something you should know about cellulite. Technically, it doesn't exist. Not in medical dictionaries or journals, and certainly not on you...The American Medical Association states flatly that there is 'no medical condition known or described as cellulite in this country." (Shape, March 1989).

If cellulite doesn't exist, why is it one of the hottest, most talked about body issues for women today?

Once I decided to write this book, I began to do research in various libraries. Cellulite is a household term among women, so I was certain I would find information in the public and medical libraries. I was shocked. I visited numerous libraries and **not one of them had a single book available on cellulite!**

At the University of California, Irvine Medical Library I found 172 books on the topic of obesity. There was not one book or even a medical journal that addressed cellulite. I did find some information in a few periodicals, but most of the articles were very superficial and inconclusive.

At first this was disappointing, because I realized that medical researchers and the AMA did not recognize cellulite as a medical problem. Then I remembered that traditional western medicine only diagnoses and treats disease and illness. Most doctors are unconcerned about cellulite, or tell women there's nothing they can do about it.

It is understandable that physicians who spend so much of their time focusing on life threatening diseases do not have the time for what appears to be only a cosmetic problem. However, preventive medicine is coming increasingly into the forefront of medical training, and it is only a matter of time until a lifestyle which eliminates cellulite and other related problems becomes a part of overall recommended health care.

My theory is based on the fact that *cellulite does not exist as a type of fat;* instead, cellulite is a condition resulting from a combination of separate, yet physically related problems. As mentioned earlier, these imbalances in the body include poor fat metabolism, possible hormonal imbalance, lymphatic congestion and other factors. The approach taken by the Anti-Cellulite Program stresses internal cleansing and a comprehensive exercise program.

GENETIC FACTORS: WOMEN ARE DIFFERENT

The fact that you are a woman automatically predisposes you to the tendency to develop cellulite. Just because you have a tendency to get it does not mean that it is a healthy, normal thing to occur on a woman's body.

There are genetic variables that cause women to manifest cellulite. Collectively these factors can lead to a lumpy, rippled appearance of the skin and flesh called cellulite. This book examines the causes, control and cure for cellulite through special attention to lifestyle.

OUR CONNECTIVE TISSUE IS DIFFERENT

The tissue located just below the surface of the skin is known as subcutaneous tissue. It is the substance which binds the skin to underlying tissue and bones. Included in this are fat cells, which vary in number and size, and from person to person. Women generally maintain a high level of fat cells in the uppermost portion of their subcutaneous tissue. In between this fat layer, fine dividing walls of the connective tissue are anchored to the overlying connective tissue of the skin.

In men, this subcutaneous tissue is much thinner and has a tighter and more compact crisscross pattern. This stronger design of the connective tissue keeps overweight men from developing cellulite.

For women the fat cells tend to bulge in an irregular fashion, causing the outer skin to look and feel lumpy. It can be compared to a cheap down comforter in which the feathers simply do not stay in their designated compartment. Instead they clump together here and there, and wherever they find fellow bed feathers.

OUR SKIN IS DIFFERENT

Women also have thinner skin than men do. The outer skin layers, termed the epidermis and corium, are more delicate. Thus they are more likely to make fatty deposits underneath visible. As women grow older, these layers of skin become less elastic and even thinner, creating an even more dimpled appearance.

That's why proper skin care is important to the external treatment of cellulite. Certain skin creams can be helpful in toning the skin, thus giving it a smoother appearance.

OUR FAT CELLS ARE DIFFERENT

The fat beneath a woman's skin tends to form into large, round, overfilled cells. In comparison, male fat-cell chambers are divided into small, polygonal units that do not bulge when filled. Cellulite inflicted areas tend to include the upper thigh area, as well as the buttocks, abdomen, and upper arms. Here, the subcutaneous tissue is composed of three layers of fat, with two planes of connective tissue between them.

As a woman's thinner tissue structure continues to thin with age, excess fat cells begin to surface. To further aggravate the problem, connective tissue walls between fat cells also become thinner, thus allowing the weakened chamber containing fat cells to bulge.

The best remedy for this problems is strength training exercise. *Fat cells are the fuel of muscle tissue.* The more muscle tissue you have, the more fat-burning ability your body has as a result. This is one of the reasons why strength training is so effective in eliminating cellulite.

15

OUR HORMONES ARE DIFFERENT

Due to their hormonal system, women have a higher percentage of body fat than men. Our hormones actually determine how much fat we carry, as well as where it is distributed throughout the body. Estrogen, the primary female hormone, ensures that women carry plenty of fat in their hips, thighs and buttocks. This fat is protective padding for babies, and begins to accumulate at the onset of puberty.

Our endocrine glands are intimately related to our moods, our weight, and our menstrual clock. Any imbalance in this finely tuned system can cause cellulite, PMS and other menstruation related symptoms often considered psychological.

Many symptoms of PMS are related to cellulite. Among these are the potential to retain water, a sluggish metabolism, as well as low blood sugar (hypoglycemia) that can cause food cravings and an increase in appetite. **A less acknowledged symptom of PMS is a temporary increase of cellulite.** This increase usually lasts until after the onset of menstruation.

Have *you* ever noticed about one week before your period, your cellulite becomes more pronounced? I have talked to many women who became aware of this phenomenon only after their attention was drawn to it.

I do not believe that either PMS or cellulite is normal. If you refuse to accept these conditions, you will begin to accept the possibility of releasing them for good. Incidentally, if you are currently suffering from PMS, you will probably notice an improvement of the symptoms as you come into a more balanced state of health during this Anti Cellulite Program

Letting go of cellulite involves much more than just losing fat. It has to do with the care and maintenance of the entire body, including the skin, organs, tissues and fluids. Cellulite can be eliminated through regular exercise, a healthy diet, skin care and internal cleansing. It is a gradual process that requires your willingness to make some changes in your life, but the rewards are both beautifying and gratifying.

OUR WATER BALANCE IS DIFFERENT

Women generally retain more water than men. Water retention can dramatically affect cellulite. The more water we retain in and around our cell tissues, the more severe and exaggerated the appearance of cellulite. Causes of water retention will be discussed in greater detail later in this chapter.

17

THE LYMPHATIC SYSTEM
and how it affects cellulite

The lymphatic system can be described as the "garbage disposal system" of the body. Its many functions include fluid drainage, detoxification, as well the transport of vital proteins, fats, and hormones to the cells. When compared to the other vessel system of the body, the blood vessel system, the lymph has twice the vessels of the blood. Unlike the blood, however, lymphatic fluid has no pump. Instead, it must rely on a mild process of contraction coming from the lymph ducts and the surrounding skeletal muscles.

While the blood is the fluid most responsible for transporting nutrients to the cells, it is lymphatic fluid that carries excess waste products out of the body. When the level of toxins is too high for the lymph to handle, it becomes sluggish and congested. This can be compared to a sink that drains slowly but is not sufficiently bothersome to call the plumber.The result is an increasing accumulation of this waste which settles in the safest possible location of the body: our fat.

Lymphatic *capillaries* actually penetrate and surround every living cell in our body. In fact, they are in great abundance in areas of the the body where blood capillaries cannot be found at all. The lymph carries nutrients to cells which the blood does not reach, in addition to carrying waste away from the cells.

18

The lymph is responsible for removing both by-products of the metabolic process, as well as the toxins that come from our lifestyle and environment. The lymph then carries these wastes to the thoracic duct and back into the blood stream, where it can be further processed by the liver and kidneys, and eventually released from the body or changed into harmless substances by these cleansing organs. The purpose of the thoracic duct is to carry the wastes from the lymph nodes and to send them into the blood stream for further processing.

If these toxins were to accumulate in other areas of the body, for example in our organs and brain, we would age and die very quickly. Although these vital tissues do accumulate some waste, toxins are more safely stored in the fat. For example, people who were exposed to high levels of DDT during and after World War II often did not experience the toxic effects of this insecticide until they had a severe weight loss. Only then was the DDT released from the fat into the bloodstream, with veteran's hospitals even reporting some fatalities. An internal cleansing program can help these poisons to be removed from fat stores more safely.

LYMPHATIC FLUID

Exactly what is the lymph? Lymph, or lymphatic fluid, is a clear white fluid consisting of white blood cells or leukocytes. **These are the warrior-cells that maintain our immune system**. They circulate throughout the entire body within the lymphatic system. They are maintained and regenerated by means of the lymphatic glands.

LYMPHATIC GLANDS

Lymphatic glands, otherwise known as lymph nodes, can be found throughout the body in clusters along the lymphatic vessel system. They are especially noticeable as nodules the size of a pea (in their healthy state), in the groin area, along the spine, under the armpit and in the throat. When the flow of the lymphatic system becomes overloaded to the point of congestion, they swell to many times their normal size.

The lymph nodes are responsible for straining lymphatic fluid. They actually clean it much like a bath cleanses the body. When the fluid returns to the thoracic duct it should already be clean from the action of the nodes. The lymphatic fluid is then sent back into circulation, and the cycle begins again.

So if the lymph is not moving properly, if it is congested with toxins, this cleansing becomes very difficult. Have you ever noticed the swelling and soreness of the small lumps in areas under your chin, under your armpits, and in your groin area? These are overworked and overburdened lymph nodes fighting valiantly against invading disease organisms. They are sore because of the irritation caused by these poisons.

Dr. Frank Chapman, an osteopath from the earlier part of this century was the first to research cellulite and its relation to the lymph. In his work, he found that when the flow of energy to the lymph system becomes blocked, specific reflex points responsible for regulating the flow of lymph fluid shut down, turning off the overloaded system. These blockages can cause enlargement of lymph glands, tenderness and pain, and eventually other chronic problems such as cellulite.

THE LYMPHATIC PUMP

Although the lymphatic system is much more extensive than the blood system, it does not have an efficient pump to help move it along. The blood can rely on the heart to make certain that it circulates throughout the entire body. Under X-rays it has been observed that the lymphatic fluid relies on a much weaker pump action to keep it in circulation. It can be termed as a 'suction pump'. Our lungs act as a vital component of this suction pump, helping the lymph to circulate.

The lymph moves in one direction only: towards the heart. For example, the fluid moves from the feet, up against gravity, towards the chest. It also moves from the head and arms downward, again toward the chest. When we inhale very deeply into the chest area, we are actually helping to draw the lymph towards our chest area, thus maintaining good pumping action.

When our breath is too shallow the movement of the lymph is impaired. This is why exercise is so beneficial to the Anti-Cellulite Program. Not only does exercise burn fat and create shapely muscles, but the increased lung action (deeper breathing) promotes better lymphatic circulation. The suction pump of the lymph becomes reactivated.

It is interesting to note that if the lymphatic system were to suddenly stop moving, death would result. The circulation of lymph is just as important as the beating of your heart.

The areas in which cellulite occurs most often are all slow circulation areas. Whenever the lymph moves against gravity, and through a low circulation area, it slows down. Like the little red engine "that could" chug up the steep hill (however with great difficulty), the lymph has a hard time moving uphill in our body.

THE
LYMPHATIC – CELLULITE
CONNECTION: MY EXPERIENCE

Once, when I was experiencing a great deal of personal stress, I drank too much coffee, and ate the wrong foods. I noticed that the cellulite returned visibly, even though I was exercising vigorously every day. Not only was the cellulite on my body more pronounced, but when I touched areas of my body where the lumps were most obvious, they felt very tender, much like a sensitive bruised area. In fact, I was able to locate the tenderness specifically to knots of tissue under the skin. These tender knots were located in the very area where the vessels of the lymph are most concentrated, although I did not know it at the time. Then my mind made the connection! *Cellulite and the lymph are intimately related!* I was later diagnosed as having a premalignant lymphatic system. The threat of cancer was enough for me to change my lifestyle drastically.

Exercise was no longer as effective in eliminating cellulite because my lymphatic system was in serious trouble. It was more than just congested. It was developing into a dangerous state of disease.

I began working with a wonderful holistic physician, Dr. Robert Gahn, who advised certain lifestyle changes and also recommended some cleansing herbal and homeopathic remedies. As my lymphatic system began to regain a healthy state, so did my energy level and vitality. Within a few months, the painful nodules and cellulite had disappeared.

It is hard to give an exact time frame for the loss of cellulite, because of the great variation of health of the individuals. My own changes, undertaken with vigor and determination, took approximately three months.

HOW BLOOD CAPILLARIES AFFECT CELLULITE

Blood is about 90% water. Within our blood capillaries, a certain amount of blood proteins can be found. The purpose of these blood proteins is to maintain a normal balance of water in the blood. It is quite normal to have a certain amount of seepage out of the blood capillaries. This seepage delivers nutrients to the cells. With cellulite this fluid seepage is apparently excessive. The dilation of capillaries contributes to the formation of cellulite.

There are three main causes for abnormal dilation of blood capillaries. The first is mental or emotional stress. The second cause is a sedentary lifestyle. Without the deep breathing caused by exercise, the whole body, including the blood circulatory system, suffers. The third cause of blood capillary dilation is poor nutrition.

THE SODIUM – POTASSIUM PUMP AND ITS RELATION TO CELLULITE

Every living cell in the body has an occurring process known as the *sodium-potassium pump*. A high level of potassium is maintained inside the cells, while outside the cells a low level of sodium is available. To experience a high level of energy within the cell, and therefore in the body, it is important to maintain a high potassium/low sodium balance. This creates an energy-producing pump action that is on-going and continuous within the living cells.

If our system has too much sodium and not enough potassium, certain complications take place in the body. We may experience water retention, hypertension (high blood pressure), heart palpitations and other more severe problems.

When an upset in this delicate balance occurs, increased sodium levels can cause a bursting of the tissue. This bursting can lead to the development of cellulite. Here's why:

The blood moves at a rapid pace. The lymph capillaries, being congested from an overabundance of waste, move too slowly. The blood then pours deposits into the tissues, and the overburdened lymph cannot keep up with this high rate of deposit. The fluid and toxins are found in such large amounts, that the system becomes imbalanced. This is one reason to keep the level of dietary sodium at a minimum, while maintaining an adequate amount of potassium in the diet.

COLON HEALTH AND CELLULITE

Unless foods are metabolized and wastes eliminated, the body cannot function properly. Constipation can aggravate cellulite significantly due to auto-intoxication (self-poisoning). Just as a clogged drain will back-up a dirty dishwater, a clogged colon pumps toxins and poisons right back into the body. The lymphatic system becomes overworked and burdened, and as a result, sluggish.

While stress can be one cause of constipation, the foods we eat play a major role in keeping one "regular". All foods in the Anti-Cellulite Diet are excellent for colon health. Keeping the inner environment clean is *key* in the releasing of cellulite.

FREE RADICALS AND CELLULITE

One of the main causes of aging and disease is also the overabundance of certain wastes in the body. These are known as *free radicals*. Free radicals are also responsible for the aging process of the skin.

On the skin, free radicals take the form of *lipid peroxides,* otherwise known as rancid fats. They are responsible for the damage to the outer membranes of the cell, which are comprised of collagen and elastin. Collagen means *to stick together,* while elastin means *elastic.* Free radicals destroy or damage these vital cell membranes, so they cannot hold tightly together. Like a wornout rubber band, the skin loses its elasticity. It wrinkles and sags. This destruction of the tissue further aggravates the problem of cellulite.

WHERE DO FREE RADICALS COME FROM?

We are exposed to an incredible amount of free radicals every day. Their sources range from a polluted environment, chemically treated water, and chemicals in our food, to the rarely considered sources such as the by-products of our own digestive process as well as poisons our bodies create under stress.

One of the reasons that too much stress can lead to sickness and disease stems from the production of free radicals by the body when it is unable to cope with mental, physical or emotional stress.

HOW TO CONTROL FREE RADICALS?

Now that we have examined the physical imbalances that cause cellulite, we can begin to take charge of those factors which we are able to control. Those currently beyond our control, such as environmental pollutants, may perhaps be changed as we choose to accept the environment as our individual social responsibility. For now, we will focus on what we can control.

An overview of the poisons around you that you can consciously eliminate include caffeine, alcohol, drugs, unnecessary medication, nicotine, junk food additives, sugar, salt, chemical pollutants at work and at home, as well as personal stress. Your goal will be to minimize these factors as much as possible. The approach is simple, practical and beneficial. The changes do not require much time, money or energy. All that is necessary is an honest inventory of habits you need to change in order to be healthier and to eliminate cellulite.

Begin by locating the sources of these toxins, whether they are in your cleaning supplies, medicine chest or cosmetics. In this book you will learn to eliminate toxins by following specific dietary guidelines and using supplements. You will also learn how to expel the toxins from your body and skin through exercise, relaxation, visualization and other techniques. As you follow through with the program, you will find that you are nurturing yourself more than you ever have before. As you feel better, you will have more time and energy for the other priorities of your life.

A MULTI – FACETED SOLUTION TO A MULTI-FACETED PROBLEM

So far you have learned that cellulite is not just *one condition* due to *one problem.* Cellulite is the result of the slowing down of several vital functions in the body. Just as it took years to slowly and gradually develop cellulite, it is a gradual process to completely eliminate it. There are many approaches one can take to the problem. If dealt with from only one perspective, the results will be only partial and temporary.

It is only by considering every facet of the problem, and in turn utilizing all available resources, that there can be a permanent and healthy solution.

The
Cellulite
Solution

Chapter 3

THE ANTI-CELLULITE DIET

BASIC PRINCIPLES

The Anti-Cellulite Diet serves one primary purpose: *to free the body of the excess wastes and fats that are at the root of cellulite.* Our aim is to eliminate foods that pollute or add excess fat to the body, and to eat an abundance of foods that are known to cleanse the digestive system. By incorporating a simple method of food-combining which speeds the transit time through the digestive system, toxic metabolic by-products will be eliminated.

Weightloss is a natural side effect of a cleansing and detoxifying diet. By radically reducing fat intake, caloric intake is reduced without the need to use a traditional calorie counter.

BENEFITS OF THE ANTI-CELLULITE DIET

WHAT TO EXPECT

After several days on this plan, you will possibly have more energy than you had before. You may also experience greater mental clarity, better sleep, and an ability to function at a much higher level. This is because your body will be freed up in its energy expenditure. It will not be so sluggish from using its energy for waste removal. The load on the lymphatic system will also be less, giving it a chance to decongest. Your body will begin to let go of cellulite much more easily.

You will still be eating three meals a day, and even be able to snack when you feel hungry. The idea is to 'eat clean'. The foods you eat will be cleansing and nourishing. The foods you will be avoiding are those that tend to increase or cause cellulite.

Following is a list of foods to focus on, Anti-Cellulite Foods, as well as foods to avoid, Cellulite-Creating Foods. Both lists are highlighted by commentaries and explanations. Although you can create your own diet plan based on this information, an Anti-Cellulite Diet sample menu is included later in this chapter.

If you are ever unsure of which foods to eat, it is a good idea to copy the Anti-Cellulite Foods Shopping List at the end of this chapter and keep it in your purse. It is a simple and easy reference chart that will come in handy when you first begin the program.

ANTI-CELLULITE FOODS

Anti-Cellulite foods are cleansing to the body, lymphatic system and also to the digestive system. These foods are also high in a variety of nutrients. They are all generally whole, unprocessed, and low in fat. In contrast, foods that lead to cellulite are more toxic to the body and tend to be high in fats, sugars, salt, preservatives and additives.

VEGETABLES: All vegetables are excellent. Avocados should be eaten in moderation since they are fairly high in fat. Fresh vegetables are best for maximum nutrition and enzyme content. Steamed vegies are next, followed by frozen, canned and pre-cooked ones.

I highly recommend seeking out a store where you can purchase fresh, *organically grown* produce. There is increasing evidence that the chemicals used for the growing and storage process of conventional produce may be harmful not only to the body but to the environment. Organically grown food is certified to be free of these poisons. This is not only better for releasing cellulite, it's better for your whole body.

FRUITS: All fruits are beneficial on this program. Fruits are also rich in nutrients and enzymes. In addition, fruit has the shortest transit time through the digestive tract. Bananas and dried fruit should be consumed in moderation (no more than one banana or one quarter cup of dried fruit per day) due to their high calorie and natural sugar content.

For optimal nutrition, fresh fruits are best, followed by frozen, canned and dried ones. Make sure dried fruits are free of sulphur dioxide.

GRAINS: Barley, millet, buckwheat, quinoa and rye are the best grains for the Anti-Cellulite Diet. These are the lightest of grains and are easiest to digest. Amaranth, oats, rice, and corn are also very good. The only grain to avoid is wheat. Many women are allergic to wheat, or tend to retain excess water after eating this grain. This is due to a reaction to the gluten in wheat. Take note of the following alternatives to wheat breads.

WHEAT BREAD SUBSTITUTES: Corn tortillas, blue corn tortillas, rice cakes, rice flour bread, rye flour bread, any bread using the above grains. Sprouted wheat bread contains no gluten and is therefore an acceptable substitute for regular wheat bread. In fact, all sprouted grain breads are both delicious and higher in nutrition than grain flour-based breads.

BEANS AND LEGUMES: Lentils, split peas, navy beans, soy beans, mung beans, garbanzo beans, pinto beans, kidney beans are all excellent. For the vegetarian, beans and legumes, in combination with grains are among the best sources of protein. These need not be eaten during the same meal to derive the complete protein benefit. As long as grains and legumes are eaten on the same day, protein intake will be sufficient.

SEEDS: Sesame, pumpkin, sunflower, and flax-seeds are acceptable. Seeds are best used as seasonings rather than snacks. Although they are high in protein and nutrients, the fat content of seeds is very high. If you are not concerned about losing fat, and only need to lose cellulite, seeds in larger quantities are fine. If soaked overnight the enzymes in seeds are put into action and the fats and other nutrients are pre-digested. *Soaked seeds* take the stress off of the digestive system, have better nutritional value, and are good to eat as snacks.

SOY FOODS: Tempeh, tofu, tofu hot-dogs, and soy milk are all high protein substitutes for animal products. While these are not yet available in most grocery stores, soy-based meat substitutes can be found in the freezer or refrigerator section of your health food or specialty store.

SPROUTS made of beans and seeds: Mung, lentil, alfalfa, clover, sunflower, and garbanzo sprouts are very rich in protein, enzymes, vitamins and minerals. Sprouts of all kinds are highly nutritious, cleansing and low in calories.

CONDIMENTS: Most condiments on the market tend to contain excessive salt, fats, additives and preservatives. For dressings and seasonings, be creative and make your own, or check your health food store. To make your own, experiment using herbal seasonings, raw sauerkraut, salsa, lemon, vinegar, and brewer's yeast.

OILS AND FATS: Small amounts of olive, canola, or sesame oils are acceptable. *Do not use these for deep frying or pan frying.* Remember, fats are best used minimally or not at all. They can be used for sauteing foods or in salad dressings.

It is said that we need only a small amount of fat in our diet. This is true. But it is also true that we can get this small amount of fat from foods that we generally do not consider fat containing. For example, spinach contains 11% fat. Vegetables, fruits and grains offer all the fat we need in our diet.

ANTI-CELLULITE BEVERAGES:

WATER:
Purified, filtered, spring, distilled, or purified carbonated water are always preferable to tap water. Distilled water is best on a cleansing diet such as this.

JUICES:
Unsweetened fruit and freshly extracted vegetable juices are very healthful. Fresh juices are best. If you are preparing your own juice, use organically grown fruit as much as possible. If you are purchasing bottled juice, check the label for sugar, salt, additives or preservatives.

COFFEE SUBSTITUTES:
Herbal teas, grain beverages, and chicory coffee are flavorful substitutes for coffee and caffeinated tea.

CELLULITE-CREATING FOODS

Certain foods are are linked to an increase of cellulite on the body. Since cellulite is due to an excess of fat, wastes and water in the body, the foods to eliminate are those which promote these. The foods on the the following list are high in fat, salt, sugar, preservatives, additives, caffeine or alcohol. Continuing to eat foods and drinks with these ingredients, you are only prolonging your cellulite problem. Avoid the foods on this list as much as possible!

FATS: All fried foods should be avoided, as well as butter, margarine, animal fats, saturated oils and fats, nuts and nut-butters. Look out for hidden fats in salad dressings, gravies, sauces, baked goods and sweets.

SUGARS: Sucrose (white or brown sugar), molasses, fructose, maple syrup and corn sweeteners are often chemically treated. If you must sweeten, barley malt syrup,rice syrup and honey are acceptable in small amounts. Check the labels of your cereal boxes, muffins and breads. Many of these products contain added sugar. An excellent alternative to sugar is concentrated fruit juice. If you avoid sweets as much as possible, you may eventually lose your taste or desire for sweetness.

WHITE AND WHEAT FLOUR PRODUCTS: As mentioned earlier, the gluten in wheat products may cause reactions such as bloating, swelling, and for some women, emotional upset. The following products are usually made with wheat: breads, muffins, pasta, crackers, cookies, cakes and other baked goods. Natural food stores and some grocery stores carry alternative products made with rice, barley, soy or rye flour. Avoid wheat as much as possible especially if you suspect you are sensitive to it.

FLESH FOODS: Pork, beef, lamb and venison are best avoided on the Anti-Cellulite Diet. Often these contain growth hormones and antibiotics injected into the animals (or added to their food) while they are still alive. In addition, meats are sometimes treated with color and other chemical substances that act as tenderizers or preservatives. The effects of these chemicals are currently being scrutinized by the FDA, and some countries have already outlawed their use.

Flesh foods also have the slowest transit time through the digestive tract. This means that auto-intoxication is much more likely.

In my opinion, *flesh foods are just not a good idea, neither for people nor for the animals!* We can get plenty of protein from vegetarian sources. Contrary to popular belief, certain vegetable foods have a complete protein content, for example spirulina and chlorella. For more on these superfoods, see Chapter Four on supplements. A well balanced vegetarian diet is highly recommended to combat cellulite. It will greatly speed your progress.

If you still choose to eat meat, moderate amounts of lean poultry and fish are acceptable. "Free range" chickens are free of chemicals. Remember to eat poultry with the skin removed, since the skin contains most of the fat. Also keep in mind that these foods are best prepared without fats. Broiling, barbecuing, poaching, steaming and fatfree sauteing are the preferred cooking methods.

The inclusion of meat in the traditional four basic food groups is for its protein content. In recent years the amount of protein considered necessary for a normal diet has been lowered.

EGG and DAIRY, O.K. in moderation:
Eggs and dairy products tend to be mucous forming and therefore can lead to mucous congestion in the body. Small quantities of nonfat milk products and egg whites are fine. The white contains no fat and has only 15 calories, as opposed to the egg yolk which is mostly fat and has about 65 calories! Low fat cheese and farmers cheese are also acceptable.

Especially avoid the following egg and dairy products: ice cream, fatty cheeses, whole-fat milk, butter and egg yolks.

CONDIMENTS and SEASONINGS:
Ketchup, relish, mayonnaise and fatty salty dressings should not be used. Look for alternatives that are sugarless, saltfree, chemical free and low in fat. Period.

Read labels; there are many products on the market today that are healthy and good to use. If you really want to get rid of cellulite, the tricky foods need to be monitored. Even though they are usually used in small quantities, they can have an orange peel effect on your hips, thighs and buttocks.

CAFFEINE: The most common sources of caffeine to be avoided on this diet include coffee, black tea, some sodas and chocolate. Caffeine can lead to a high level of toxicity in the body. In addition, it can be a great burden to the lymphatic system and the central nervous system.

If you consume large quantities of coffee, do not stop your habit all at once. This could lead to withdrawal symptoms such as headaches, irritability and dizziness. A better way to stop the coffee habit is to ease off of it gradually. Every day lower your intake by about a half cup. This way your body has the opportunity to come back into balance more gradually. Many women are also addicted to diet pills. This may be linked to the high levels of caffeine in these products.

SALT: Although most people are aware that excessive salt in the diet can lead to water retention and other problems, few people pay much attention to their salt intake unless they have a major medical problem. However, some of the burdensome weight on your hips and thighs can be released by cutting out the salt. This doesn't mean just disposing of the saltshaker; it means doing some serious label-reading.

Almost all prepackaged food contains salt, especially chips, crackers, canned and frozen foods, as well as baked goods. If you don't have time to do your own saltfree cooking, many healthfood stores carry saltfree chips, canned goods and other foods. So look out for salt, salty seasonings, soy sauce, tamari sauce, and processed foods containing salts.

Excellent salt substitutes include herbal seasonings, powdered kelp (which can replace the salt in your shaker), vinegar and spices. As you gradually lower your consumption of salt, you won't even miss it.

ARTIFICIAL SWEETENERS:
Artificial sweeteners have always been controversial. Because there is no concrete evidence that any of the artificial sweeteners on the market are completely safe, they should be avoided on this program. In addition, you are training your tastebuds to crave healthier foods, not sweet foods.

The bottom line is that artificial sweeteners are not whole foods. They are synthetic chemicals that have no business in a healthy, organic body.

ADDITIVES AND PRESERVATIVES:
Prepackaged and prepared foods are often loaded with additives, coloring agents and preservatives. People are so concerned with wanting their food to look pretty, they don't care whether the ingredients might be causing cellulite, cancer or other health complications.

42

Just about every unnatural, manmade substance in and on our food is potentially dangerous. Our bodies do best with whole and unprocessed foods.

Read labels! Be aware of what is being put in America's meals. There's a reason for calling it junk food. Many of the additives stay in your body longer than you may think! Cellulite is born of toxins and fats. Look out for them. Be a label warrior. Read, learn, and be aware.

ADDICTIVE SUBSTANCES: The addictive substances to avoid include alcohol, cigarettes, abused prescription drugs, "recreational drugs", sugar and caffeine. These not only cause cellulite, they poison your body.

The body is simply not equipped to deal with these heavy toxins on a daily basis. The more they build up in the body, the worse cellulite becomes. It's that simple. Use this program to get these substances out of your life and out of your system. In fact, if you follow the diet, supplement and exercise suggestions, you will be detoxifying the buildup of these chemicals, and helping them to exit your body.

ANTI-CELLULITE FOOD COMBINING

You may be eating all the right foods, but combining them in a way which leads to toxins in the body, and therefore cellulite.

Symptoms of gas, indigestion and incomplete absorption of nutrients are some of the effects of poor food combining.

Many people already know about and follow food combining guidelines for the purpose of better digestion and increased energy. A lesser known benefit is the elimination of cellulite.

I attended a women's business meeting one morning at a local restaurant. I observed some of the breakfast selections these women had made. I noticed that most of them had ordered oversized plates of ham, eggs, buttered toast and hash browns. Most of these women were also very fat. Sitting to my left was a slender young woman who had ordered a fruit bowl, just as I had. I asked her if she was practicing food combining. She smiled and mentioned that she was about to ask me the same question. This woman went on to tell me that she was approaching age 30 and had just given birth a few months ago. She said the only way she was able to maintain her cellulite-free figure, was by adhering to the principles of food combining.

FOOD-COMBINING PRINCIPLES

The foods we eat move at different speeds through our digestive system. Fruits move through quite rapidly, followed by vegetables, grains, legumes,fats and flesh foods.

Food is digested in the stomach by means of our digestive juices. For each type of food, the stomach produces specific digestive juices. In other words, different juices are secreted for different foods. It is quite possible that when eating certain foods together, the corresponding digestive juices can actually compete with each other. They can actually neutralize the effect of one another. Some examples of improper combining are meat and potatoes, chicken and noodles, cheese and bread, cereal and milk.

Do you notice a pattern here? These combinations all represent the combination of carbohydrates and protein. Proteins and starches do not digest together well in the stomach. When these foods are eaten in one sitting, the transit time of the food is decreased, causing the food to putrefy in the digestive system.

Proteins are derived from animals (including all flesh and dairy foods), as well as legumes, nuts and seeds. These foods demand a digestive juice that is especially **acidic** in nature.

Carbohydrate foods include breads, grains, pastas and cereal. These are digested by means of an **alkaline** digestive juice.

Basic chemistry tells us that by nature of their properties, acids and alkalies neutralize each other. This makes it difficult for the body to digest a starch and protein at the same time.

What is it that causes funny noises and discomfort after a large meal? Since the food cannot easily move through the digestive tract, and it does not have the strength of the stomach's digestive juices to prepare it for the small intestine, it remains in the stomach for an abnormal length of time and eventually ferments and putrefies. This difficult and incomplete digestion releases toxins into the system which manifest as cellulite.

To keep the food moving through the digestive tract as efficiently as possible, adhere to the following guidelines.

FOOD COMBINING GUIDELINES

1. Only eat fruit with fruit. "Eat 'em alone or leave 'em alone". No vegetables, starches, proteins or other foods should be eaten with fruit.

2. Carbohydrates (grains, breads, pastas) may be eaten with any vegetables, but not with proteins or fruits.

3. Proteins (meats, legumes, seeds, nuts) may be eaten with vegetables, but not with starches or fruits.

IT'S SIMPLE. The best way to acquire these habits is to practice them for at least three weeks. Do not judge the effectiveness by anything you hear or read. Even if you don't agree with them, following them cannot harm you. After three weeks, judge your results. Take note of any differences in your energy level, digestion, and especially cellulite. In the Appendix, you will find a food combining chart that lists examples of the food groups. Also, check the sample menu to give you an idea of the principles in practice.

Food-combining works. It works for good health, good digestion, and it works in eliminating cellulite. Eating foods in a specific manner will help decrease fluid retention, flush excess toxins out of the system, and most importantly, help to reduce cellulite.

SAMPLE MENU

BREAKFAST
fresh fruit bowl
herb tea

LUNCH
baked potato or yam stuffed with
steamed broccoli
fresh vegetable salad topped with
low-fat salad dressing

DINNER
vegetarian chili
steamed cauliflower and sweet peas
small dinner salad

THE ANTI-CELLULITE
SHOPPING LIST

The following list is a composite of the foods you will be eating on The Anti-Cellulite Diet. You can find most of them in the produce section of your grocery store. Remember to look for certified organically grown whenever possible. Also, if you know of some exotic fruit, vegetable, grain, seed or legume that is not listed here, keep in mind that if it's a whole food and low in fat, it's an Anti-Cellulite Food! You have the author's permission to photocopy this list for personal use. Take it with you during the first three weeks of the program.

Fruits:

     Apples
     Oranges
     Strawberries
     Apricots
     Kiwi
     Grapes
     Bananas
     Peaches
     Pears
     Plums
     Grapefruit
     Nectarines
     Papaya
     Blueberries
     Blackberries
     Tangerines
     Fresh figs
     Mango
     Cherries

Vegetables:

     Carrots
     Broccoli
     Lettuce (and other leafy greens)
     Beets

Cabbage
Asparagus
Peas
Artichokes
Summer squash
Sprouts
Cucumber
Tomato
Green beans
Peppers
Celery
Kale
Turnips
Cauliflower
Mushrooms
Spinach
Radish
Onions

Root Vegetables (starches):

Potatoes
Yams
Sweet Potatoes

Grains and Flours (starches):

Barley
Millet
Kasha (buckwheat)
Quinoa
Rye
Brown or White Rice

Amaranth
Kamut
Corn Meal
Oat

Cold Cereals (starch):

Nutrigrain (rice or corn)
Oil-free, sugar-free granola
Puffed rice
Puffed millet
Puffed corn

Hot Cereals (starch):

Oatmeal
Cream of Rice
Cream of Rye
Kasha (cooked buckwheat - this is not considered to be wheat!)
Any cooked grain except wheat

Pasta (starch):

Rice Pasta
Corn Pasta
Kamut Pasta
Quinoa Pasta
Any non-wheat pasta

Beans/Legumes (Protein):

Lentils
Split peas
Navy beans
Soy beans
Mung beans
Garbanzo beans
Black beans
White beans
Kidney beans
Lima beans
Pinto beans
Black eyed peas

Soy-based foods (protein):

Tofu
Tempeh
Soy milk
Tofu hot dogs
Tempeh burgers

Seeds (protein):

Sesame seeds
Poppy seeds
Pumpkin seeds
Sunflower seeds
Flax seeds

Beverages:

Pure water
Herbal teas
Fresh fruit juices
Fresh vegetable juices
Sparkling flavored mineral waters
Grain beverages (coffee substitutes)

DETOXIFICATION

When given the opportunity, the body will cleanse and heal itself. By following this type of diet, your body's natural cleansing properties are improved. It clears out wastes, regains lymphatic health and reduces its fat levels. *You may experience some discomfort due to detoxification or psychological withdrawal.*

PHYSICAL CLEANSING SYMPTOMS

Physical discomfort may be experienced as a result of the change in your lifestyle. You may have some mild cleansing reactions that indicate your body is releasing toxins. This is uncomfortable at first, but is actually a *positive sign.* Your body is utilizing its newfound energy to pool toxins that have accumulated in your body. They temporarily circulate in your bloodstream and lymph, and are then flushed out of the system entirely.

If you are already eating well and exercising, you will probably not experience any symptoms. Only those making drastic changes in their lifestyle will experience these cleansing effects. Among the most common are irritability, dizziness, white coating on the tongue, sleepiness or flu-like symptoms. The flu symptoms can include elevated body temperature, nausea and tender skin. These are a positive indication that your lymph has been very toxic, and is now taking the opportunity to clean out.

Remember: *do not be alarmed!* After a few days you will feel much better. You are doing your body a favor and your efforts will not go unrewarded.

FEAST DAY

Often when a person begins a limiting or restricting diet, they will do wonderfully for a period of a few days, and sometimes even a few weeks. Then, 95% of the time, this discipline takes a 180 degree turn for the worse, and the behavior changes to rebellion. This sometimes results in a binge that leaves the dieter in as bad or worse shape than before. The focus will shift to the consumption of salty, fattening junk food, as if to make up for lost time.

When I was dieting very vigorously at the onset of my strength training program, I had a rule for myself: I allowed myself one

Feast Day a week. I kept my diet full of whole, nutritious foods, and never ever ate salty, fatty, or junky food. But one day a week, usually on a weekend , I would allow myself to eat whatever I wanted. This is an excellent way to deal with any desires for foods that are a temptation. Whenever a craving comes up, just tell yourself: "Wait until Saturday and have it when you go out to dinner." By Saturday you might not even crave that food anymore!

It's simply an emotional relief to know that you're not stuck on your diet forever. You will no longer feel rebellious about being on any diet program and one day of this will not affect your long-term results on the program. Feast Day will ultimately give you more staying power in the long run.

Chapter 4

THE ANTI-CELULITE
EXERCISE PROGRAM

BENEFITS OF EXERCISE

Exercise is a fountain of youth. You will see the difference on the outside and feel the difference on the inside. Everything changes. Your skin takes on a fresh glow, your resting heart rate decreases, your blood pressure normalizes, and the circulation of the blood and lymph improves.

Improved circulation means increased nutrient transport to every living cell of the body. It also means a cleaner, better flowing lymph. A better flowing lymph cleanses and discards of the toxins which create cellulite more efficiently.

You may also notice that your moods will be better. This is because your body creates powerful and beneficial drugs, known as endorphins as a result of regular exercise. More potent than any available antidepressant, these mood elevating chemicals will provide you with the positive mental fuel to propel you to higher levels of success.

ANTI-CELLULITE BENEFITS

A balanced, lean and contoured body is the overall result of a balanced exercise program. Such a program focuses on strength training (using free weights), cardiovascular training (aerobic exercise) and flexibility training (stretching). All three of these approaches are used in the Anti-Cellulite Program. However, *my main purpose in writing this book is to introduce you to the type of exercise that makes the greatest difference with cellulite: strength training.* The cellulite ridden body that you see now will be transformed into a beautiful and toned physique practically before your eyes.

Although the exercise portion of this program may present the greatest challenge for you, if you will stay with it for a minimum of three weeks, you may never want to stop. You will already be looking much better and you'll be surprised at how much your cellulite will already have been reduced.

STRENGTH TRAINING: THE ANTI-CELLULITE EXERCISE OF CHOICE

Strength training is the exercise of choice in fighting cellulite. So powerful is this approach to exercise, that it can literally reshape and contour your body in the matter of a few short months.

Men have known about weight training for a long time. Women have generally shyed away from weight equipment, opting for aerobics classes instead. Only in the last decade have a small number of women learned to work out with weights and weight machines.

To get a visual image of the results this type of workout program can yield, procure a copy of Joe Weider's *Shape* magazine. Most of the models in this magazine use a **complete workout** approach. The bodies of these women are lean, firm and free of cellulite.

There is a magical result that occurs with a good weight training program. The contours and shape of the body can be transformed by the exercises you choose. You are in control of how your body looks, and you can guide the process by choosing the right type of exercise: strength training.

It is so simple. The results come faster than with any other exercise. Yet if this exercise is so incredible in combatting cellulite, why aren't more women doing it? Why am I surrounded mostly by men, not women, in the weight training room?

Many women have the impression that weightlifting will make their body become large and muscular like a man's. But *unless they take steroid drugs or use extremely heavy weights no such thing can ever happen.* Why not? Because women lack the hormones to make them very muscular. Fortunately, for those of us who enjoy looking like women, we are just not designed to be super-muscled!

STRENGTH TRAINING: MYTH VERSUS FACT

Testosterone is the hormone crucial to building muscles. Estrogen is the hormone responsible for maintaining higher fat levels in the body. Men and women have both of these hormones in their bloodstream. However, men have much more testosterone in their blood, with just a trace of estrogen, while women have more estrogen, with just a trace of muscle-building testosterone. This low level of testosterone in a woman's blood stream is why she will never build large, masculine muscles. For her, weight training is just a means to a stronger, leaner physique.

Many of the professional female bodybuilders who are muscle-bound take the testosterone hormone to muscle them up. Even after heavy workouts and drugs, most of them are still very feminine. Our goal is not to be muscle-bound, but to be lean, healthy, toned and fit. Our goal is to release cellulite from our bodies forever.

Cellulite interupts the feminine line of the body. Strength training brings back the beautiful curvalinear shape that is natural to a woman.

Strength training is the foundation of this program. It will make 90% of the difference for you. If you join a gym in your area, it may be helpful to find a personal trainer to help you through the initial workouts, so you are certain to use correct form. Community Colleges and Public Parks and Recreation centers also often provide classes. If you are working out at home, check the Appendix for the home gym equipment you will need.

ANTI-CELLULITE AEROBICS

Aerobic exercise has long been recognized as the best fatburning exercise. At a moderately low intensity we can encourage our body to burn subcutaneous fat, and thereby to release the very substance that is at the heart of cellulite. This means that our fat cells will shrink and the cellulite will become much less visible.

Aerobic exercise, however, can never help us get rid of cellulite without the addition of strength training. We need to build more of the very stuff that will take the place of the fat we are burning: muscle tissue. This is not to be confused with the false assumption that fat turns into muscle. Aerobic exercise may help tone our muscles, but since we women have inherently very little muscle, strength training with free weights is the best approach for creating shapliness.

By definition, aerobic means "with oxygen". This means that the exercise uses large quantities of oxygen. For those interested in burning fat, this is the most beneficial type of exercise. Our goal is to increase the capacity of the heart-lung system to deliver blood, and thereby oxygen to the working muscles during sustained exercise.

Aerobic exercise also serves some very important functions in the Anti-Cellulite Program. It conditions the respiratory and circulatory systems which directly increases the capacity of the lymphatic pump. Improved circulation and respiration mean improved perspiration. This means that we will be able to use another system our wonderful bodies have for waste elimination: sweat. The skin is the largest cleansing organ we have, and perspiration is a means of excretion of toxic substances through it.

HOW TO BURN CELLULITE AND FAT MOST EFFICIENTLY

As mentioned earlier, aerobic activity, at a moderately low level is the fastest way possible to burn fat. I often see women storming their way through an incredibly vigorous aerobic workout. If their goal is to burn fat, they are working much too hard.

Studies show that the most effective exercise for weightloss is aerobic movement below target heart rate for 20-60 minutes at least three days per week. If your goal is to burn fat along with the cellulite, it is important to include this type of activity in your workouts.

Although many kinds of activities are aerobic, the best exercises for fatburning purposes are those that are rhythmic and continuous in movement. Also, low or non-impact activities are best for preventing injuries. Following is a list of some of these. Since I do aerobic exercise seven days a week, I constantly change the exercises to keep interested and motivated.

Rhythmic, continuous movement aerobic exercises include:

* Walking
* Bicycling
* Rebounding (trampoline)
* Skiing
* Low-impact aerobic classes
* Rowing machines
* Stair-climbing

It is especially important to chose an activity that you enjoy. For those who are not generally prone to injury, high impact aerobic activities are also excellent. People who engage in high-impact aerobics (jogging, jumproping, high impact aerobic classes) should be aware of the absolute necessity of at least a ten minute warm up period before doing the high impact activities.

PRIMING THE FAT PUMP

Another fatburning technique has been termed: Priming the Fat Pump. Priming your fat pump requires that you feed your body a small amount of carbohydrate food before your workout. For example, eat an apple, a piece of bread or a muffin.

This will direct your body's energy system to use its own bodyfat as a main source of fuel. If you work out in the morning on an empty stomach, without any carbohydrates, your body burns muscle tissue for its fuel. So make sure to eat your carbohydrates to prevent this. You will also experience an additional increase in endurance and an energy boost.

ANTI-CELLULITE STRETCHING

Flexibility is vital in maintaining body mobility, preventing injuries, *and* staying free of cellulite. Stretching exercises are more beneficial to the lymphatic system than any other form of exercise, opening congested areas, and allowing for a better flow of the lymphatic fluid. Once again, toxins can more readily be transported out of the body.

Stretching is also a wonderful stress releaser. Much of the waste in our bodies is created within our very own body by emotional stress. When we set aside 5-15 minutes during the day to stretch, we can help let go of tension and muscle constriction.

As with strength and endurance, flexibility varies widely among individuals. Women are generally much more flexible than men. This is one of the benefits of having less muscle. Lifestyle has a tremendous effect on our flexibility. Those of you who wear high heels are likely to have more of a problem with flexibility. Sedentary or overweight individuals tend to be less flexible as well.

A marvelous way to incorporate stretching into a daily routine is to learn yoga. Yoga not only feels wonderful, but it is extremely beneficial in releasing blocked energy. This can help improve organ function, and bring balance and health to tired, overburdened lymphatic and endocrine systems.

BEFORE YOU GET STARTED

It is best to have a physical examination before beginning any regular exercise program, especially if you are thirty or more, and you have not had an exam lately. This will give you an idea of your overall physical condition before you start. An examination also protects you against any potential problems that could surface from the exercising.

If you are suffering from a chronic disease such as arthritis, osteoarthritis, asthma, obesity or coronary heart disease, your workout will do much more than reduce cellulite. Indepth scientific research has shown that these chronic diseases improve dramatically with regular exercise. However, do consult with a physician before beginning the program.

Remind yourself to begin slowly and gently, allowing your body to become accustomed to exercise. This way you will experience only mild muscle soreness and will be more likely to continue with the program. You can progress into a more vigorous workout gradually.

THE COMPLETE ANTI-CELLULITE WORKOUT

Often people choose one type of exercise, feeling they have found their niche, and therefore neglect other exercises from which their body might benefit. For example, if a woman decides upon stretching as her chosen form of exercise, she may improve her flexibility, but still feel exhausted after a long walk or jog. A person who enjoys regular aerobic-type activities may be in excellent cardiovascular shape, but have difficulty carrying heavy grocery bags from the car to the kitchen. There are those who have discovered strength training and can easily carry their heavy groceries, yet have trouble touching their toes. For maximum benefit all three areas should be developed.

For A Lean, Strong And Flexible Body Exercise Aerobically, With Weights, And By Stretching.

You don't have to become a super athlete to create your perfect body. In an hour or more a day, three or more days a week, you can do it all. The right combination of exercises can do wonders for your physique.

The best workout is the one that leaves nothing out.

Discover what it takes to melt into your ideal body, the one you were meant to have in the first place.

EXERCISE FLOW CHART

Here's a flow chart for your workout schedule. Of course you may exercise longer than the designated time; I've just listed the minimum workout for the maximum improvement.

5" Aerobic warm up. Slow, rhythmic activity.
15" Higher intensity aerobic exercise.
35" Strength training with weights or Nautilus equipment.
5" Stretching exercises.

= 1 HOUR OF EXERCISE.
MINIMUM: 3 DAYS PER WEEK.
OPTIMAL: FIVE DAYS PER WEEK.

NOTE: If you find that you want to exercise longer, an increase in the aerobic and strength training sessions will speed your progress even more.

BEGIN WITH A WARM UP

A few years ago, participants of aerobic classes, runners and other fitness enthusiasts routinely warmed up with stretching exercises. This practice has now been abandoned and is considered possibly dangerous. The purpose of a warm up is literally to warm up your muscles and joints. This means bringing blood to the muscles and senovial fluid (lubricating fluid) to the joints. *Light, rhythmic aerobic movement, such as walking or jogging in place is an ideal warm up,* while stretching is most effective when the muscles are already warm. However, stretching is excellent after a vigorous aerobic session.

The warmup includes getting the heart rate from a resting rate to over 100 beats per minute.

YOUR AEROBIC WORKOUT

Following the warm up, the next fifteen minutes are devoted to high intensity aerobic activity, including those mentioned earlier in this chapter. The heart rate is ideally brought to and kept at target level which can easily be calculated. Your heart rate is important because it tells how hard you are exercising. By learning to check your heart rate, you can measure the ideal level of intensity for your workout. Techniques for checking the pulse and heart rates are found in the Appendix.

As the aerobic workout burns fat, it is also an excellent warm up for the more strenuous portion of your workout: the strength training. Following the prescribed progression of exercises can greatly reduce the risk of injury to your joints and muscles.

YOUR STRENGTH
TRAINING WORKOUT

The strength training workout is the third step, and it specifically aims at cellulite reduction and makes this program different from other exercise programs. It can be done at home or at a local gym, at a Community College, or Parks and Recreation facility. If you live near a gym, I highly recommend signing up for a membership there. It provides an atmosphere away from home where you can be around others who also want to feel better and take care of their bodies.

The gym is a kind of get-away for the day, as well as an opportunity to meet like minded people. Fitness oriented people are usually friendly, confident and offer a good support system.

WHAT EXERCISES TO DO FOR STRENGTH

While cardiovascular exercise can be done every day without physical difficulty, strength training is best divided into a schedule that allows recovery for individual body parts. For example, instead of exercising the entire body with weights every day, it is best to choose certain days for certain body parts. This gives the body an opportunity to recover and develop while you exercise other areas. For a three day a week strength training program, the following schedule is recommended:

DAY 1: CHEST AND TRICEPS

Bench Press
Incline Dumb Bell Press
Cable Flies
Decline Dumbbell Press

Triceps Pushdown
Triceps Overhead Press
Triceps Dips

DAY 2: BACK AND BICEPS

T-Bar Rows
Dumb Bell Rows
Lat Pulldowns (wide grip)
Seated Rows

71

            Biceps Cable Curls
            Biceps Preacher Curls
            Biceps Incline Dumbbell Curls

DAY 3:   **LEGS AND SHOULDERS**

            Squats
            Lunges
            Leg Extensions
            Leg Curls
            Calf Raises

            Shoulder Dumbbell Flies
            Military Press
            Shoulder Shrugs

EVERY WORKOUT DAY:
Abdominals and Buttocks

            Crunches
            Oblique Abdominal Curls
            Leg raises
            Donkey kicks
            Buttock squats

Each exercise should be done for a minimum of ten repetitions and three sets. Begin at this level, and as you become stronger, increase either the weight or the number of sets.

There are many different types of workout programs. There is no "best" except what works best for you. The one I suggest is great for beginners, and not enough for those who are already fit. For example, I exercise five to seven days per week. I spend at least thirty minutes on the aerobic portion and an additional hour or more in the weight room.

Because of the importance of doing these exercises correctly, the how-to-dos are not included in this book. A competent trainer is familiar with all of the standard techniques and will supervise your learning and performance of them. Bring this list to a trainer at your gym, or acquire a workout manual, such as the ones on the Recommended Reading List in the Appendix. I especially recommend Joyce Vedral's book: Now or Never.

THE COOL DOWN: STRETCHING

It is safest to stretch *after* working out, when the muscles are warm. Stretching is a wonderful way for the body to cool down after the main exercise portion of your workout.

When done correctly, stretching places the muscles in a position that promotes elongation of the muscle. You should feel some discomfort, but no actual pain.

Flexibility is essential for preventing injuries due to exercise. Inadequate shoulder flexibility, for example can lead to rounded shoulders. This in turn can lead to lower back pain, due to overcompensation of the back muscles. Basically, when the muscles are tight due to tension or misuse, stretching is a relaxant par excellence.

Here is a brief list of some of the most effective stretching exercises. Please refer to a personal fitness trainer, or Bob Anderson's book Stretching for a more detailed description of individual exercises.

If you are already familiar with some basic stretching positions, use them as a starting point to begin your routine now.

5-10 Minutes of Feel-Good Stretches:

> Hip flexor stretch
> Quadriceps stretch
> Hip adductor stretch
> Hamstring stretch
> Shoulder extensor stretch
> Low-back stretch
> Calf stretch
> Straddle stretch

To improve flexibility, it is best to stretch a minimum of five days a week. To maintain the same level requires three or more days a week. In our routine, it is best to choose 8-10 positions, and hold them for what is known as a *static stretch*. This means that the position will be held, without bouncing, for a minimum of 20 seconds. Bouncing can lead to injury or soreness. Hold the stretch to the point of discomfort, but not pain.

INJURY GUIDELINES

If you choose to engage in high intensity aerobics or work out with heavier weights, it is very important to be aware of any warning signs your body may be giving you. If you listen to the small pains, you may be able to save yourself greater discomfort, money and especially recovery time. Remember that an injury could mean a setback in your workout program. Time off will only delay results, and can lead to frustration.

Be aware of any signs or symptoms that persist for more than three to five days. Pain, swelling or movement impairment are common indications that you should ease up on your workouts until the affected area is completely recovered.

Given a chance, the body will heal itself; however, the constant irritation of an injury by exercise can lead to permanent damage. The basic message is: *listen and respond to your body!*

JUST DO IT!

Make the time to take the most important step in this program and **begin to exercise**. Make it your homework *right now* to join a gym or set up your own home gym. Then get going. If the information here has sparked a desire in you to begin a complete exercise program, ACT ON IT!

75

Chapter 5

ANTI-CELLULITE TECHNIQUES

EXTRAS THAT CAN MAKE THE DIFFERENCE

Most of the techniques included in this chapter have to do with topical stimulation of the skin, and/or the detoxification of the lymphatic system. Each treatment is unique and beneficial, and every practical application in this book is interdependent. Whether it be diet, exercise, supplementation or any of the techniques in this chapter, each will decrease cellulite to a limited degree when used alone. However, if you are committed to eliminating all of the cellulite on your body, permanently, it is vital that these techniques be used in conjunction with the rest of the program. The results will be complete, and much more permanent than any "crash program".

77

THE LOOFAH

The loofah is a naturally fibrous plant that grows on a vine. It is harvested, dried, and is often used as a feel-good, scruffy bath and shower sponge.

Women can directly benefit from using the sponge on cellulite-covered areas. The scruffiness gives the skin a circulation boost, as well as a gentle lymphatic massage. This brings more oxygen and nutrients to the fatty areas of the body where circulation tends to be slower. It also assists the lymphatic system in removing and disposing of toxins more quickly.

Since the loofah absorbs water fairly easily, proper care of it will help it last. It should be taken out of the bath or shower to dry. If it remains in areas of high moisture, it will disintegrate and mildew in a matter of days.

DRY BRUSHING

Dry brushing is a specific application of the common skin brush. Most commonly used to remove dead, dry skin from the surface of the body, the skin brush, used correctly, is beneficial in helping the lymphatic system to move in the proper direction. It should be done when the skin is dry, for example before bathing or showering

As you may recall from Chapter Two, the lymphatic system has a more extensive network of capillaries than the blood system, yet it has no direct "pump" to help circulate. It relies mostly on muscle movement and good respiration, appreciating any help it can get. The lymph moves in only one direction: towards the heart and lung area This is the direction to follow when brushing the skin.

Very lightly and gently brush from your toes, up your legs, up your torso, to your chest. Then brush from your hands, up your arms, and towards your heart. Finally, very gently brush your face, down your neck, and again towards the heart area. This process should feel invigorating. Although it is sufficient to do this once a day, twice a day is ideal. You may actually feel your lymph circulating more freely throughout your body as a tingly sensation.

Dry skin brushing also removes dead skin cells and gives the skin a more youthful, glowing and resilient appearance.

FINGER BRUSHING

If you do not have a dry brush, or find the sensation of it too rough for you, the same process may be done with your finger-tips. Using the same directional flow as with the brush, gently and quickly brush your finger tips along your skin towards your heart. This is an effective technique in helping the lymph reach its destination. The process is even beneficial when done with clothing on. The lymph is very sensitive and will benefit from the attention. Finger brushing is also a light, pleasant self-loving massage.

NEURO-LYMPHATIC MASSAGE

Special lymphatic massage points are primarily located on the back, thighs, chest and head. These points may be massaged for 10-30 seconds with moderately deep pressure. If you are doing the massage yourself, you can locate them by palpating areas of your chest and head, and reaching your hand to your back area and touching along your spine.

You may feel a ticklish or tender sensation when these points are touched. This lets you know you've found them. After you've touched on them once or twice, your fingers will automatically know where to go. The sorest points are usually the ones most in need of massage. The function of the massage is, again, to increase the flow of lymphatic fluids that may be blocked or moving sluggishly.

If you regularly visit a massage therapist, mention these special points. They can then focus and concentrate for a few extra minutes on these areas. In fact, most certified massage therapists are aware of the importance of the lymphatic system and will understand how to use massage to constructively reduce cellulite.

WHOLE BODY LYMPHATIC MASSAGE

Many holistic health professionals and massage therapists offer whole body lymphatic massages as one of their services. It is a whole body massage that concentrates on massaging the entire lymphatic system. This is a wonderful and enjoyable way to get rid of cellulite.

For best results, lymphatic massage should be performed on a regular basis, at least once a week, and should be used in combination with the other self-help techniques. You may want to remind your practitioner to focus on the neuro-lymphatic points mentioned earlier and areas in which cellulite is a problem.

ORIENTAL HEALING ARTS

ACUPUNCTURE:
Acupuncture is an ancient Chinese healing art that can help bring the body back into a state of balance. By inserting special needles in specific acupuncture points, energy is released in areas of the body where the flow of energy had been blocked or constricted. With regular treatments (at least once a week), acupuncture can effectively help the body to release cellulite.

81

CUPPING:
Chinese massage therapists use this method to heal pain, speed recovery and to draw toxins from the body. The process involves heating cup-like devices, and allowing them to create a heat-induced suction on certain areas of the body. They are left in position for a period of twenty or thirty minutes. This breaks up stagnation in the area (energy, blood, fats, water, etc.).

SHIATSU (Acupressure):
Shiatsu is a type of Chinese massage based on acupressure points. Massaging these points along the entire body can greatly assist in the reduction of cellulite by allowing freer circulation of energy. This means better lymphatic and blood flow as well as improved organ function, all beneficial in detoxifying and restoring balance to the body.

THE BENEFITS OF YOGA

Although flexibility was discussed in detail in Chapter Five, yoga is an approach to stretching that is unique. I chose to include it in this chapter because it should not be considered as part of a vigorous workout. Done once or twice per week, yoga can help the anti-cellulite process in many ways.

There are many kinds of yoga, all of which originated in India as an integral part of the Hindu religion. Hatha yoga is the kind with which Americans are most familiar. It combines asanas (postures) which strengthen and stretch the muscles, with breathing and sometimes with spiritual or meditative techniques. Although yoga does not play a direct role in the removal of cellulite, the gentle persistent stretching of the muscles contributes towards relaxation and unblocking of energy.

Yoga is said to unblock energy in the body. Blocked energy may be a contributive cause of dis-ease and cellulite. These blocks are physical tension, usually stemming from emotional and mental tensions. Most physicians and physical therapists recommend these exercises in varying degrees for people of all ages. Many communities offer yoga classes, or at least a list of yoga instructors. There are also some excellent yoga video taped programs that you can practice in the privacy of your home. As in the case of weight training, a disadvantage of an audio or videotape is the lack of correction and unsupervised practicing.

Some women use their age and past childbearing as an excuse to live with cellulite. But it doesn't need to be that way! No matter what our age or background, cellulite is only a temporary condition that can be eliminated with proper diet, exercise and state of mind. For example, E.J. McVay, a noted yoga instructor and psychotherapist, does not have a trace of cellulite on her fit body. She is thirty-six years old and has two children. Although she attributes her lack of cellulite mostly to her healthy vegetarian diet and positive mental/spiritual outlook, she feels that her disciplined commitment to yoga is most responsible for her youthful and beautiful physique.

MINERAL SALT BATHS

In Europe, physicians include prescriptions to visit mineral bath spas as a part of a medical treatment. European medical insurance often covers most of these spa visits! These are not vacations, but carefully supervised and regimented treatments attended by homeopathic and allopathic physicians, registered nurses and licensed physio-therapists.

There are spas for various medical conditions. Many of them are mineral bath spas at which the water is ingested in controlled amounts and also used topically by bathing. Thus the dosage is carefully controlled.

Why are these baths considered so beneficial? It must be more than the warm water in these spas that has such a healing effect on the body. Mineral salts are said to have a strong detoxifying potential. Some have the ability to draw poisons from beneath the skin. After such a bath a person often feels rejuvenated and the skin becomes very soft and silky.

You need not spend a fortune to obtain the same benefit. In the United States, bath shops or healthfood stores carry "earth mineral salts" or "mineral hot spring salts". These have been collected from spa sites, dehydrated,and packaged for use in the bath tub!

Chapter 6

ANTI-CELLULITE
SUPPLEMENTS

NUTRITION FOR THE BODY:
Inside and Out

Supplements for the Anti-Cellulite Program include food supplements as well as special skin care products that can help you towards achieving your goals. The nutrients and herbs listed can usually be found in health food stores or in specialty stores. **Pure water, vitamins, minerals, herbs, amino acids** (proteins), **"super-foods"**, special **body-wraps, bath salts** and nutrient-rich skin **lotions** or **creams** can all benefit you. They provide nutrients that assist the body in detoxification, circulation and weight-loss.

Although none of these products (except pure water) is required on the Anti-Cellulite Program, they may accelerate your results.

87

The effects of some of them are cosmetic and not curative. Who's to argue that looking good and feeling good won't motivate you to continue following the program?

Our main source of nutrients should be fresh, whole foods, as Mother Nature intended. However, with the soil (and therefore our food) as depleted and chemically treated as it is today, it seems sensible to supplement your diet with vitamins and minerals. Herbs can also be very helpful in bringing the body into its own natural state of balance, without being forceful. Amino acids are the building blocks of life, and individually serve many specialized functions in the body.

This program is not intended to have you binge on vitamin pills. Excessive water soluble vitamins are eliminated in the urine and overdosing on certain fat soluble vitamins can be harmful. Americans have the reputation of having the most expensive urine in the world! Instead, choose your primary focus for this program, for example weight-loss, detoxification or metabolism balance, and choose the appropriate supplements accordingly.

WATER:
THE ANTI-CELLULITE BEVERAGE

The benefits of drinking water are almost endless. We will only focus on those benefits specifically helpful in eliminating cellulite. Water will be your most important "supplement" on this program. Six to eight (8 oz.) glasses a day is a healthy quantity. It is important that the water you drink be clean, and not full of chemicals often found in tap water. For instance, while fluoridated water is intended to prevent tooth decay, if you drink tap water in large amounts, you may be getting too much flouride, thus putting an additional burden on your body's cleansing system. At this writing many cities are questioning their fluoridation programs for precisely this reason.

WATER DETOXIFIES

Water is vital for weightloss and cellulite-loss. Not only does it assist in nutrient transport, but it flushes the toxins out of the body that have been collected by the lymphatic system.

During periods of weight loss and detoxification, the body has much more waste to dispose of. For example, all of the byproducts of fat metabolism and lymphatic cleansing need to be removed from the body. The more excess fat a body has, the greater the metabolic waste products. This is why the heavier person on a weight loss program needs more water than the thinner person.

WATER IS THE BEST DIURETIC!

That theory sounds backwards, doesn't it? It would seem that people who retain excess water in their bodies should drink as little fluid as possible. But the less water the body receives, the more it will fight to hold on to every drop consumed. It slips into survival mode, thinking it will need to retain a backstock in case of drought. This could save your life if you were ever deprived of fluids. But since there is no drought, you should give your system as much as it requires.

Some people abuse diuretics, and often do more harm than good. The swelling they experience in their feet, hands, legs, buttocks and breasts is only temporarily removed. After the effect of the diuretic has worn off, they will probably retain even more water.

The most natural and healthy solution to water retention is to give your body plenty of water, and to eliminate excess salt. That's all. If you happen to indulge in excess salt, just drink extra water that day. The water forces excess sodium through the kidneys and out of the system.

WATER IS A NATURAL APPETITE SUPPRESSANT

Many weightloss programs such as Weight Watchers recommend drinking an eight ounce glass of water before every meal. They suggest that when hunger pangs are especially strong, simply drinking enough water will subdue the desire for food. This simple suggestion is as effective as it is safe.

Don't drink ice water before, during or after meals. The cold will cause contraction of the ducts and inhibit enzymes from entering the digestive tract, thereby slowing digestion.

WATER GIVES YOUR MUSCLES TONE AND YOUR SKIN RESILIENCE

About half the weight of muscles comes from water. It gives them the ability to contract and prevents dehydration. Drinking water also improves the appearance of facial and body skin by keeping it hydrated, thus keeping it from sagging. This is beneficial against both cellulite and wrinkles.

ANTI-CELLULITE HERBAL SUPPLEMENTS

Herbs are foods that are highly concentrated in nutrients, volatile oils and trace substances which can improve health. They have been used for thousands of years to assist the body in healing, or to relieve symptoms and pain due to chronic conditions.

In combating cellulite, herbs can be used both topically, as compresses or body wraps, and orally as tablets, teas or tinctures. Certain herbs can increase circulation in specific areas of the body, and also improve skin tone and strengthen connective tissue. Herbs can prove beneficial in helping the body to release toxins as well. They are often helpful to internal cleansing programs. The following is a list of herbs that I found particularly helpful during the Anti-Cellulite Program.

Gotu Kola is recognized primarily for its potential to balance the metabolism of the connective tissue. Taken orally or used topically, gotu kola can noticeably enhance connective tissue structure. Benefits include a softening of the skin, improved blood circulation, and a decreased feeling of heaviness in the legs.

Escin is a special herbal compound extracted from the seed of the horse chestnut. Taken orally, its properties include the ability to strengthen capillary walls, act as a mild diuretic and as an anti-inflammatory. Escin can also be beneficial when applied topically in compresses or skin creams.

Butcher's Broom can be used effectively for the treatment of cellulite by taking the herb orally as tea, capsules or tinctures, and also by means of its topical application to the skin. Butcher's Broom is also popular for the treatment of varicose veins, hemorrhoids, and inflammatory conditions.

Bladderwrack is a seaweed which is often found in cosmetics and cellulite treatment programs. It is most recognized for its soothing and softening effects on the skin. The topical application of this sea algae is excellent in the treatment of cellulite as a body compress or added to bath water.

Ginseng is an adaptogenic herb containing 42 vitamins and minerals including germanium, calcium and iron. It has been proven to increase circulation, strengthen the body's immune system and stimulate energy within the body. Some cultures use it as an aphrodisiac. Siberian, Chinese Red Panax and American are among the most popular.

Red clover has been used as a strong blood purifier and cleanser. It is possibly the best herb for the cleansing of the lymphatic fluid and glands. It is delicious as a tea, but can also be taken as a tincture or tablet.

ANTI-CELLULITE AMINO ACID SUPPLEMENTS

Proteins comprise approximately half of a cell's dry weight and are found in every part the living cell. Hormones, enzymes, blood-clotting factors and anti-bodies are all types of proteins.

Proteins can be described as the building blocks of life. In turn, amino acids are known as the "building blocks of protein". Proteins are composed of amino acids, which are very simple molecules. They differ from fats and carbohydrates in that they contain nitrogen. Each amino has its unique molecular structure, and based on this structure, it serves its own unique function in the body.

In an isolated, or pure form, we can use amino acid supplements to target particular nutritional goals. We can choose specific amino acids to promote faster muscle growth, more efficient fatburning, better memory retention, and even allergy relief.

There are over 24 known amino acids some of which are particularly beneficial for the Anti-Cellulite Program.

L-Carnitine assists in the regulation of fat metabolism. Especially helpful to the liver, heart and skeletal muscle, l-carnitine serves as a carrier for the transmission of fatty acids into the mitochondria, where the fat can be burned as energy. In overweight people, fatty acid metabolism has been shown to improve with l-carnitine supplementation.

L-Cysteine is a powerful detoxicant of environmental pollutants, especially heavy metals. Long term digestive imbalances can be the result of toxicity from foods, beverages and inhalants. Heavy metals can be "chelated" (bound) by l-cysteine and then flushed from the body. L-cysteine has extremely reactive sulfur-containing bonds that have an attraction for these metals. They are literally locked up by cysteine and then eliminated from the body. L-cysteine works well with Vitamin E and Selenium to offer cellular protection from dangerous free radicals.

L-Methionine is a lipotropic, fat emulsifying amino acid, which assists the breakdown of fats. Along with l-cysteine, this amino has highly reactive sulfur-containing bonds which have the ability to detoxify and remove metals from the body. L-methionine also aids in the maintenance and health of the liver and digestive system.

L-Threonine is also a lipotropic aid that promotes good liver function. L-threonine is important in the Anti-Cellulite Program due to its ability to help manufacture cellular membrane lipids, as well as collagen and elastin.

L-Taurine is a byproduct of l-cysteine. This amino acid produces taurochloric acid, known to increase bile flow, which is essential to the metabolism of fat.

ANTI-CELLULITE VITAMINS

Vitamin A maintains healthy skin, digestive and urinary systems and vision. It is necessary for the synthesis of steroid hormones and immunity cells.

Vitamin C helps to form and maintain collagen. In a strong, healthy body collagen has the consistency of a stiff jelly, much like gristle or tough gelatin. Collagen is the cement that holds together the cells of the body.

A deficiency of vitamin C, however, allows this tissue to break down. Although many diseases can result from this type of deficiency, cellulite is one of the less health threatening effects. Why? Because collagen keeps our cells united! Cellulite is due to an excess of fat, water and toxins contained by weak connective tissue.

Vitamin E is generally recognized as the major lipid (fat)-soluble anti-oxidant. This vitamin is helpful in protecting the tissues from free radical damage. Stephen Levine, expert of free radical/antioxidant nutrition, notes that chemicals which are foreign to the body may damage our cells, and especially the liver during the detoxification process. This damage can be mitigated by supplementing with vitamin E.

Vitamin B-6 is a natural and safe diuretic. B-6 is also vital to amino acid metabolism.

Choline and Inositol are components of the B-vitamin family, These nutrients are extremely effective in assisting the body in its production of lipotropics, and therefore the metabolism of fats. In combination with vitamin B-6, these nutrients serve an important function in reducing bodyfat and cellulite.

ANTI-CELLULITE MINERALS:

Chromium is often termed GTF (Glucose Tolerance Factor) Chromium. It is an essential mineral for carbohydrate metabolism. It can be helpful to those individuals suffering from hypoglycemia by assisting proper insulin production. Chromium has also been shown to be helpful for weight-loss.

Selenium is often referred to as "the antioxidant mineral". In combination with vitamins C and E, it is an excellent free-radical scavenger. It can therefore be a great help to your detoxifying process. The toxins released during this process will be easier for your body to dispose of with the help of this mineral.

Germanium may be taken for the strengthening of the immune system. It is also a possible catalyst in supplying oxygen to living tissues. Since our surface immune system is primarily our lymphatic system, germanium can greatly benefit the reduction of cellulite.

Zinc is vital to the metabolism of carbohydrates, alcohol, and fatty acids. Zinc is also crucial to healthy immune (lymphatic) function, and is necessary for the proper function of the reproductive organs.

"SUPERFOODS"
and other helpful supplements

Acidophilus is a variety of Lactobacillus bacteria that establishes a healthy intestinal environment. It is excellent for the maintanance of colon health, and also helps in the production of B vitamins in the intestines.

Aloe Vera has been used since biblical times for both internal and external curative and preventative remedies. A desert cactus plant, aloe vera can be added to creams to improve skin tone, and consumed as a beverage for internal cleansing and rejuvenation.

Bee Pollen is often used by athletes, peak performers and dieters for endurance, energy and stamina.

Chlorella is at least 60% protein, and is also high in chlorophyll, germanium, vitamins and trace minerals.

Spirulina, a blue-green algae, is similar to chlorella, although it is higher in beta-carotene and other trace nutrients. Spirulina is generally less processed than chlorella, and due to its natural spiral structure has maximum availability of nutrients.

Guar gum is a colloid and binding agent. It has been shown to lower blood fats by binding them in the digestive tract.

Pysillium seed is an excellent source of fiber, acts as an anti-mucoid and is cleansing to the colon.

Bioflavinoids are co-factors of vitamin C. Bioflavinoids assist the body in the production of collagen and healthy blood vessels.
They may also be helpful in combatting capillary fragility.
Beta carotene has often been termed "pro-vitamin A". It is a water-soluble non-toxic form of vitamin A, and is a highly beneficial antioxidant.

Gamma Orzanol is an anticarcinogen with lipotropic (fatburning) properties. Gamma-Orazanol is derived from rice.

Octacosanol is the active ingredient in wheat germ oil, and can help increase endurance and stamina by boosting the oxygen uptake of the body.

Inosine promotes the manufacture of ATP (energy source within the cell) in the body. It has also been found to increase strength when taken before workouts.

Co-enzmye Q10 is a fat soluble, electron-carrying coenzyme which occurs naturally in the brain, heart, liver and lymph. It also possesses powerful anti-oxidant and energy-production properties.

GLA Gamma Linoleic Acid is necessary for the production of the body's chemical messengers known as prostaglandins. Prostaglandins are essential to the production of female hormones and thereby can be helpful in reducing symptoms of PMS and cellulilte. It may be taken in the form of Oil of Evening Primrose.

LIPOTROPIC ('fat-burning') SUPPLEMENTS

Webster's dictionary defines lipotropic as "promoting the physiologic utilization of fat." The following is a list of supplements which are known to have lipotropic characteristics. They aid in the prevention of excessive fat accumulation in the body and exert a positive influence upon the intestinal tract and liver.

> CHOLINE (elemental is more powerful than bitartrate),
> INOSITOL
> CHROMIUM
> (as chromium picolinate or nicotinate)
> L-CARNITINE
> L-THREONINE
> L-METHIONINE
> L-TAURINE
> GAMMA-ORZANOL

NUTRIENTS THAT BENEFIT THE LYMPHATIC SYSTEM.

The following nutrients are best taken only if the lymph is swollen or sore. You can tell by lightly rubbing the area under your jaw or under your armpits. If it's tender, or the glands are larger than the size of an almond, the following supplements can be beneficial.

> BETA-CAROTENE (Pro-Vitamin A)
> VITAMIN B COMPLEX
> VITAMIN C
> GERMANIUM
> PURIFIED WATER
> RED CLOVER
> CO-ENZYME Q10
> ZINC

ANTI-OXIDANT NUTRIENTS

Anti-oxidants are substances which have been found to provide protection against free radicals. Free radicals are toxic compounds in the body that have the power to destroy living cells and tissue. Many people supplement their diet with anti-oxidant nutrients in order to protect their bodies from the effects of environmental pollutants, rancid fat intake, alcohol, smoke, and other carcinogens. According to research, most physical aging is due to free radical damage.

In our polluted world, it is important to protect ourselves from free radicals. The best protection against free radical damage is to lead a healthy lifestyle. In addition, it may be helpful to find a supplement containing a variety of antioxidants, such as the ones listed:

VITAMIN B-1
VITAMIN B-5
VITAMIN B-6
VITAMIN C
VITAMIN E
SELENIUM
ZINC
GERMANIUM
L-CYSTEINE
L-METHIONINE
GAMMA-ORZANOL

ENERGY/WORKOUT SUPPLEMENTS

A large number of supplements are available to increase the feeling of energy in the body. Many of these, though claiming to be "natural" can be depleting to the body and may often contain caffeine. The following supplements are not only safe, but are also helpful in delivering extra oxygen to the muscles and brain. The herbs and superfoods on this list are highly concentrated in trace vitamins an minerals which provide additional nutrients for the body as well.

BEE POLLEN
CHROMIUM
(as chromium picolinate or nicotinate)
GERMANIUM
L-CARNITINE
GAMMA ORZANOL
OCTACOSANOL
CHLORELLA OR SPIRULINA
INOSINE
GINSENG
CO-ENZYME Q10
GOTU KOLA

COLON CLEANSING SUPPLEMENTS

Although by following the Anti-Cellulite Diet you should be getting sufficient cleansing fiber from the foods you eat, the following supplements are concentrated sources of fiber. Psyllium and guar gum can be helpful by cleansing the colon. They can also benefit dieters by creating a feeling of fullness. See the individual descriptions of these items for more detailed descriptions of the benefits of each of these.

PSYLLIUM SEED
GUAR GUM
ACIDOPHILUS
PURIFIED WATER
FRESH FRUITS AND VEGETABLES
(Providing cleansing fiber, enzymes and a spectrum of nutrients)

SKIN CREAMS

Any cream or lotion will help to smooth dry, rippled skin. However, certain ingredients in a cream can help make it much more effective against cellulite. For example, the addition of antioxidant nutrients or special herbs can be beneficial in strengthening connective tissue. This can aid both circulation and elasticity.

Many anti-cellulite products on the market contain some of the following nutrients. The following herbs and vitamins can be helpful in a cream or lotion:

Vitamin A
Vitamin E
Selenium
Elastin
Bladderwrack (or other seaweed extract)
Lemon Peel
Rosemary
Aloe Vera
Escin
Gotu Kola

HERBAL BODY WRAPS

Certain herbal wraps can be excellent treatments for the temporary release of waste through the skin, as well as for toning and improving the skin's elasticity. Beneficial ingredients include the ones listed on the skin cream list.

QUESTIONS AND ANSWERS ON SUPPLEMENTS

HOW MUCH TO TAKE?

Dosages for the listed supplements will vary based on potencies and individual need. Your nutritionally minded, or holistic physician will be able to help you with this. Otherwise follow indications on supplement labels.

HERBAL SUPPLEMENTS . . . ARE THEY SAFE?

Used in moderation, the herbs listed are not only safe, but are healthy and especially beneficial in eliminating cellulite. Herbs can be considered as **super-potent foods**. They are often used in assisting the body to safely regain its natural state of balance. Many of the herbs listed can be used to make delicious teas.

SO MANY SUPPLEMENTS. . . HOW DO I KNOW WHAT TO TAKE?

It is best not to use too many supplements at once. Not only would it be more expensive to purchase a bottle of every item listed, but if your kidneys and liver are not in good condition, it could be a burden to process all of these concentrated nutrients.

I suggest that you consult with a holistic physician or M.D. trained in preventive medicine. Let them know what your goals are, show them the list of supplements, and let them help you determine the supplements that would be best for your body.

Some of the more advanced holistic health offices offer a service that can test supplements for you individually. The doctor can do a simple test that checks for compatability as well as effectiveness. Before you have even opened the bottle it can be determined electromagnetically whether this particular product will be helpful and compatible with your system. This can save you time, money and confusion.

You could also tune into your own sense of well being. If you are experiencing a lot of tenderness in the lymph nodes, you will want to concentrate on supplements for the lymph. If your diet has been unhealthy or imbalanced, you may only want to supplement with a multi-vitamin/mineral formula.

Make sure your vitamin/mineral supplement is from natural sources. Most drug store brands tent to be synthetic and bound with coal tar. They also often contain shelac as well as varnish. This would only add to the level of toxicity in your body, and make it more difficult to eliminate the cellulite-producing substances. Although many pharmaceutical firms make quality controlled products, my personal philosophy is that natural source or food bound vitamins are not only easier to assimilate, but may also contain unknown as well as known factors.

If obesity or high body-fat is a problem for you, the lipotropic aminos, vitamins and minerals would probably be best for you at this time. These will help to burn subcutaneous and intramuscular fat at a higher rate, especially if taken prior to exercise.

Instead of buying each nutrient individually, the easiest and least expensive route would be to purchase "special formula" supplements. For example, your local healthfood store should carry a selection of multi-vitamin/mineral formulas, lipotropic aids, anti-oxident formulas, etc. Check the label to make sure it includes as many of the anti-cellulite nutrients as possible.

WHAT IS THE SOURCE OF FREE FORM AMINO ACIDS?

The best free form aminos available are produced by a natural process known as the Microbiological Fermentation Crystallization Process(MFCP). These amino acids are grown in a biologically active nutrient culture which is composed of black strap molasses, glucose or beet sugar. Isolating these amino acids into their "free" form allows for the best possible assimilation of these nutrients by the body.

Other, lower quality amino acids are taken from milk or egg protein, which are inferior only because they are more difficult for the body to utilize.

HOW ARE AMINO ACIDS BEST UTILIZED BY THE BODY?

Amino acids require specific B-vitamins and minerals for complete and proper assimilation and utilization by the body. In addition, amino acids in their free form require no digestion, and can penetrate the stomach lining almost immediately after consumption. They are best taken on an empty stomach, or at least with foods which do not contain proteins. Since vitamins and minerals are required to help the aminos do their specific jobs, following them with a well-balanced meal, about half an hour later, is a good idea.

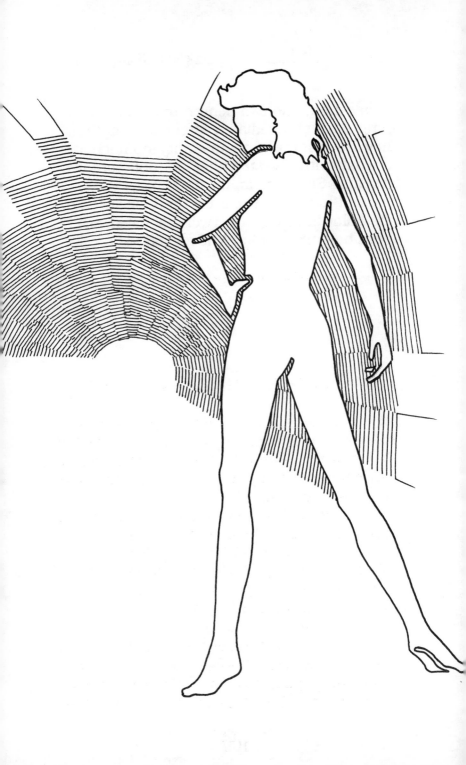

Chapter 7

ANTI-CELLULITE MIND POWER

TAKING CHARGE OF YOUR LIFE

In order to begin important and meaningful changes in your life, you need to be consciously aware of who is determining the course of your life.   What does this have to do with cellulite?

Cellulite is a symptom indicating that you may not be doing everything that needs to be done to take care of your body. Some aspect of your health care is being neglected. All you need to do is to use your body consciously and with care, as outlined in this book.

This is a chapter to come back to again and again. You may not begin to make all of the Anti-Cellulite changes at once. But once you change your thoughts and begin to open your mind to the changes that are possible, you will be much more responsive to the other guidelines of this program.

The mind is very powerful once focused upon a goal and plan of action. The possibilities are boundless. *The process of change becomes easy once your goal and purpose are vivid in your mind.*

THE POWER OF CREATIVE IMAGERY

The use of mental imagery can become an art. Your mind can be used to improve your health, finances, relationships and personal appearance. Practiced consistently and systematically, this can be fundamental to the Anti-Cellulite Program. It may actually determine how successful you will be.

The Western world is by tradition goal oriented. Although goal-setting is an excellent method to achieve one's dreams and aspirations, people often fall short of their expectations. Why does this happen?

When setting a specific goal, you need to have a **mental and emotional acceptance** along with that goal. You need to do much more than merely decide upon what you want to achieve. A part of your mind needs to imagine and accept that your desired results have already happened for you. This can be done through the use of creative visualization.

112

The purpose of creative visualization is to work through any resistances to success by using a positive approach. Instead of dwelling on the problem of cellulite, you will be focusing on your total end result. You will practice mental techniques using creative visualization and positive self talk.

RESERVE JUDGEMENT FOR THREE WEEKS

Dr. Maxwell Maltz, in his book <u>Psycho-Cybernetics</u> suggests that we reserve judgement for at least 21 days when beginning a program which requires a change in habits. He says that it requires about 21 days for old mental images to dissolve while new ones begin to jell.

In beginning the Anti-Cellulite Program, I highly recommend a commitment to the change in lifestyle for at least three weeks. During this trial period keep reminding yourself: "It's only for three weeks, that is all that is required of me". Tell yourself: **"I want my goal enough to give this program a chance"**. Initially it will be much easier for you to stick with the program. If you follow the guidelines you will see very encouraging results on your body during this time. Should temptation arise, one technique is to remember the AA adage: One day at a time.

113

Since this is the recommended amount of time necessary to acquire a new habit, and also sufficient time to notice visible results, after three weeks your mind will begin to accept these new habits as natural.

Every day that you practice the guidelines in the Anti-Cellulite Program you are improving on the progress from the previous days. You are not only creating positive results and changes in your body, you are building a mental foundation for yourself as well. You are creating a new, healthy lifestyle based on positive habits and you are proving to yourself that you are able to change or do anything you consciously choose!

The information in this chapter recognizes the fact that your mind has two distinct components: the **conscious mind** and the **subconscious mind**. While it is the conscious mind that we are most aware of during our waking hours, past thoughts and feelings are stored in the subconscious mind. Many of the decisions you make are determined by embedded memories of the past. You can create new habits of thinking, feeling and acting by reprogramming your subconscious mind with creative visualization and positive affirmations about yourself.

ANTI-CELLULITE BENEFITS OF VISUALIZATION

The almost immediate benefits that you will realize as a result of persistent and consistent visualizing include:

* Increased confidence and self esteem.

* An increased ability to stick with the program.

* An ability to go beyond limiting thoughts and feelings.

* A winning self-image at a deep, not just superficial, level.

* The body's ability to respond much more quickly to the Anti-Cellulite Program.

The mental techniques in this chapter are designed to stimulate your subconscious mind to harmonize with a new "model image" of how you truly want to look and feel. You will be programming your brain and nervous system to accept fresh images with which to identify.

115

HOW I DISCOVERED
CREATIVE VISUALIZATION

I began using the technique of creative visualization when I was sixteen years old. My mother brought home a wonderful tape by Dr. Emmit Miller that guided the listener through a relaxation process which was followed by a self-improvement section. I used the tape for both stress reduction and violin performance.

Not only did I enjoy listening to the tape, but I experienced less stress, and also began feeling more comfortable playing my violin for an audience. As this had been a challenge for me in the past, I became very interested in this technique, simply because the results were so profound.

In the past, my success seemed to be dependent on the "outer world". But it was this inner game that actually changed my perspective and ultimately the results in the "outer world".

FORM FOLLOWS THOUGHT

Einstein discovered that matter and energy are interchangeable. They are one and the same, and constantly in dance with one another. This is true about the world around us, in the area of science, and it is applicable to our personal lives as well. Our bodies are not just composed of substance. They are composed of **matter** and **energy**. These are constantly inter-relating and working together. It makes sense, then, that **our thoughts and feelings influence our physical bodies.**

Overweight people who fail on one diet after another are often holding on to heavy thoughts and feelings about themselves, or they subconsciously use the weight for protection or other psychological payoffs. The body responds incredibly well to thoughts. If our thoughts are heavy and sluggish so will the body be. Form follows thought. The body is only responding to what we hold in our consciousness.

MENTAL CAUSES OF CELLULITE

Louise Hay, in her popular book: You Can Heal Your Life, suggests that every physical ailment is linked to a probable thought/feeling. Chapter Thirteen, named 'The List', is a composite of physical problems along with (probable) mental causes. This probable cause is then followed by a "New Thought Pattern" which is a suggested positive thought that may be affirmed to oneself in order to overcome the original negative thought. Here's what she writes about cellulite:

117

"Problem: Cellulite.
"Probable Cause: Getting stuck in early childhood pain. Holding onto the lumps and bumps of the past. Difficulty in moving forward. Fear of choosing your own direction."
"New Thought Pattern: *I forgive every one. I forgive myself. I forgive all past experiences. I am free.*"

Does this sound applicable to you? If so include it in your Anti-Cellulite Program by repeating the New Thought Pattern to yourself every day. Louise Hay's results with this list have been very successful. Her book goes hand and hand with any wholistic health program. In fact, I highly recommend this book to any person making any positive changes their life.

She suggests that we take responsibility for our condition, so we can then *do something about it* . Then she has the reader repeat: "I am willing to release the pattern in my consciousness that has created this condition", and follow it with the recommended positive thoughts.

WE HAD NO PROPER MODELS

"As within, so without." This simple maxim so well illustrates that who we are today is the result of the thoughts we have been accepting since birth. Especially in our youngest years, what kind of models did we have? Who was programming our minds?

Are we unquestioningly following the same lifestyle patterns as our mothers and grandmothers? Did they portray a picture of radiant health and vitality for us into their later years? Probably not. People did not have the knowledge of proper diet, exercise, and health habits that we have available to us today.

We did not have good models. Nobody told us! Nobody showed us how to be healthy and feel good about ourselves. Look at some of the women in our society. How many women do you know who are lean, healthy, radiant and free of cellulite? Personally, I don't know many. And the ones I do know are usually the ones who exercise and practice a healthy lifestyle.

It's up to us to be the new models. We are paving the road. We will be the ones to show future generations that beautiful women are created by beautiful thoughts and a healthy lifestyle.

ANTI-CELLULITE MIND-POWER EXERCISES

Begin this program with a clear strong impression of how you want to look. Determine your ideal weight, and what you want your measurements to be. These are the components of your Anti-Cellulite goal that you need to consider. Only you can know what is ideal for you. Every woman has her own standards and ideals. Remember to make your goals realistic. If you have a strong, solid build, then a Twiggy image is not realistic for you. In fact, you could do your body damage if you tried to achieve this.

Work with what you have. Realize that you are already beautiful. Your body is the product of every thought, action and experience you have ever had. It is important to love and accept your body *the way it is right now.* Your body has been your very best friend, and no matter how you've abused it, it has continued to serve you faithfully. Make the positive changes by thanking and nurturing it for all that's it's done for you.

Begin with a list of the changes you want to make and when you intend to start. The following exercises are helpful tools that you can use both before starting the Anti-Cellulite Exercise Program, and during the course of the program. They are intended to provide positive motivation during the entire course of achieving your goal. Enjoy these and be creative with them by adding your own variations.

EXERCISE #1: SETTING YOUR GOALS

Sit down with paper and a pen and begin to make a chart of the following:

1. Your current weight/ideal weight

2. Current measurements/ideal meas urements: Include measurements of your arms, chest, waist, hips, buttocks, thighs and calfs

3. A workout schedule, or the time you are willing to commit to exercise

4. A specific, realistic date by which to achieve your cellulite-free physique

The purpose of this exercise is to make a commitment to yourself. You can go a step further by *typing out* these goals and then signing and dating the paper. Treat it like a contract with a client. You are the client, and the payoff is the rewarding experience of the new body you've created for yourself with the accompanying good feelings.

EXERCISE #2:
ANTI-CELLULITE BODYMAP

1. Select two or three magazines with photographs of women that you find attractive and physically ideal. Page through these magazines, and begin to select and cut out full body photos of women you find especially well proportioned and representative of your ideals.

2. On a large piece of good quality paper, make yourself a collage of how you ideally want to look. Use as many pictures as you desire, however remember to stick with the photos that show the whole body. Try to show front, back and side views, so as to offer a three dimensional image to your mind.

3. Leave space on the bottom of your bodymap to write in your goals, and the date by which you want to achieve this ideal.

4. Place it somewhere that it is visually accessible, for example on the bedroom wall, inside the bathroom door, or on the refrigerator. You want to see it often, so you will be reminded of what you are working towards every day.

The purpose of this exercise is to help your mind get in touch with a detailed image that you have created for yourself of what you want. Remember we are trying to stimulate your brain in every way possible, giving it pictures, images and suggestions to accept a fresh impression of what is possible for your own body.

EXERCISE #3: VISUALIZATION MEDITATION

This next exercise is an in depth practice of mental imagery. If you find it difficult at first, refer to your bodymap often. It will reinforce images in your mind, and the visualization meditation will be much easier for you. In addition, you will find it most effective to make a cassette tape of the directions. You can also order a tape of this guided visualization from the order form in the back of this book.

Sit or lie down in a comfortable position. Breathe deeply, focusing on the breath moving in through your nose, filling your chest and diaphragm area, and then moving slowly and effortlessly out your mouth. Now let all the tension drain from your body and mind, slipping out, moving easily through your feet and finger tips. Feel the tension leaving your body. Good.

As you relax even more deeply, begin to visualize a light centered in your heart. It's a small light, the size a candle flame, and you're watching it grow, slowly and gradually.

123

It penetrates your every cell. You feel its warmth radiating from your heart, into the trunk of your body, moving into your legs and arms. Now the light is filling your entire body. Feel it tingling in your fingers, where the tension had once been. You feel the liquid warmth throughout your entire body. It feels so relaxing. In fact, you are more relaxed than you have ever been.

Now say to yourself: "The light that is now filling my body is transforming my every cell. I can feel its warmth raising my metabolism, burning fat and calories faster and more efficiently. I feel its penetrating light dissolving the toxins and the cellulite that do not belong in my body. I feel myself becoming more toned, healthier and vitally alive. My body is powerfully dissolving all unhealthy substances.

My lymphatic system is flowing perfectly, easily and naturally. This radiant healing light is clearing any and all cellulite on my hips, thighs, buttocks and abdomen. I feel cleansed and purified entirely. It feels so good to be healthy, lean and strong. I am taking excellent care of my wonderful body."

Now breathe even more deeply. Feel yourself on the edge of a deep sleep. Count five breaths, and now repeat these series of words in your mind or out loud five times:

Trim. . . . . .Lean. . . . . .Free of cellulite

Forever. . . . . .Healthy. . . . . .Beautiful. . . . .

Toned. . . . . .And so satisfied with my body.

As you repeat these words to yourself, it is very important that you feel, with emotion, the wonderful feeling of having achieved your goal. You are there happy, content and satisfied with what you have achieved.

Now breathe deeply, and count yourself back to a fully conscious state, feeling refreshed and revitalized. One. Two. Three. Four. Five. Wake up! Fully aware and awake!

The purpose of this exercise is to offer your body a transforming energy to facilitate detoxification and raise your metabolism. Special attention has been given to develop the feelings that go along with having accomplished your goal. These are further enhanced through the repetition of positive affirmations.

EXERCISE # 4:
THE NAKED MIRROR

Stand unclothed in front of a full length mirror. If you don't have one, get one. This is a powerful technique. You'll need about 10 minutes for this exercise.

125

Look at your body in the mirror. *DO NOT JUDGE IT.* Just look at it. Notice your beautiful feminine curves. Turn to the side and the back, and see it as it is right now. Then take a good look at your bodymap. Look at the blue print you created for your body.

You are redesigning your body. It is already beautiful and lovable, you are only providing it with the finishing touches. To keep the plan vivid and alive, look at what you are working with, and then shift the focus to your *creative* mind.

Now close your eyes, and imagine you are still looking in the mirror. Turn from side to side. Only this time what you are seeing is your blueprint body. Your body appears to you as fit, toned, healthy and free of cellulite. You feel so good. Get in touch with the true essence of what it feels like to have completely achieved your goal. Not just on the physical level, but also on the inner, feeling level.

EXERCISE # 5:
ANTI-CELLULITE SELF-TALK

The thoughts you have about yourself throughout the day are just as important as the images and feelings you carry with you on a subconscious level. Many people aren't fully aware of the thoughts they are thinking during the day; the mind chatter is constant. For many women, this talk is negative and self-punishing. The thoughts they have been programmed to think from early childhood on, are keeping them in a less than winning state of mind, thus keeping a joyful life literally a thought away.

Imagine the changes you could bring about if all of your self-talk was positive and creative! Affirmations are positive thoughts used to reprogram the mind. Negative thoughts may be replaced by their positive opposites. Following is a list of affirmations to write or say to yourself.

AFFIRMATIONS TO ACCEPT AND TAKE CARE OF YOUR BODY

* **I love myself exactly as I am, right now.**

* **Everything I do adds to my health and beauty.**

* **Everything I eat increases my health, beauty and fitness.**

* **The more I love myself as I am now, the more beautiful and radiant I become.**

* **I am now slender and attractive.**

* **I am now free of cellulite forever.**

* **I now only desire the foods that give me more aliveness and beauty.**

127

* I enjoy exercise!
* It is safe for me to be slender and beautiful.
* I now accept the healthy, cellulite-free body within me.
* I deserve to have a toned, slender, cellulite-free body.
* I treat my body with love and care.

AFFIRMATIONS TO REPROGRAM YOUR BODY

You can actually stimulate your metabolism and speed it up or slow it down. You can help your body to release toxins and excess weight with the most powerful force on earth: your mind. If repeated on a daily basis, in a state of meditation, or just before going to sleep, your body chemistry can begin to adapt to these thoughts.

* My body is dissolving cellulite, automatically, now.
* My metabolism is burning an extra 200 calories a day.
* I am experiencing much more energy and aliveness every day.
* My body is moving toward better and better health with each breath.

* I am now breathing fully and freely,
* My body responds beautifully to exercise.
* When I sleep, my body works easily and efficiently to re lease toxins.
* My lymphatic system is circulating freely and perfectly.
* All excess water and fluids leave my body.
* My hips, thighs and buttocks are becoming leaner, more toned, and free of cellulite.
* I am feeling better than I have in my entire life.

EXERCISE # 6:
MODEL VISUALIZATION.

So far, each exercise has required that you set aside a certain amount of time to focus on what you want. Most people lead very busy lives, and may only have time to use one or two of the recommended mental exercises. Model visualization is something you can use throughout the day, and is especially helpful during times of low motivation.

When you make your bodymap, look for a specific model. This should be a woman with a build similar to yours, with the difference being your model is already fit and free of cellulite. She will be your model trainer. She is your coach. Every moment of every day on this program she will be guiding you, motivating you and advising you on your diet and exercise routine.

In your mind's eye, your model will sit down with you at meals and help you become aware of which foods are best for you. She will be certain you make it to the gym, and once you are there, she will guide you through your workout. You will not skimp on your workouts, because your model trainer will ensure that you put in your time on the exercise bicycle and help you through your last set of biceps curls.

Best of all, she is so enthusiastic about exercise and health care that it's contagious. You feel elated and incredibly happy about taking such good care of yourself. If ever you feel that you need support, you can close your eyes, relax, and ask your model trainer for help. You are very receptive, because you know that she will give you sound advice. You feel great comfort in her guidance and friendship.

This is a mental game which is very effective. If you take the time to create a vivid model guide, this technique can take you through times of doubt or confusion. Instead of heading for the refrigerator when you're feeling low, take a moment to listen to your model trainer. If you find yourself cheating on workouts, you can remember that your model trainer is watching and persuading you to push a little harder and see it through.

The guidance is actually coming from within you and your imaginary model is that part of you that really does know what is best for you. Often we are not in touch with the wisdom we already have inside of ourselves, and the model trainer can help us find our inner wisdom and surrender to it.

Chapter 8

THE COMPLETE
ANTI-CELLULITE PROGRAM

BEGINNING AND MAINTAINING
A NEW WAY OF LIFE

Contrary to what you may think, it is not a full time job to follow all the suggestions in this book! With a little planning, this entire program should fit easily into your normal schedule and budget.You don't need three weeks at a special spa to reach your goals. You can begin by following the basic foundation of the program. Then simply add as many of the self-care applications as you feel comfortable with.

The best approach to the Anti-Cellulite Program is to consult a flow chart. As with the flow chart in the Anti-Cellulite Exercise chapter, this will provide a general outline of the most important procedures to follow throughout the day. You can add to it, or change it according to your needs, but the basic structure should remain unaltered. If the core program is adhered to, then choosing from the additional techniques and varying them will not only help to counteract the cellulite, but will keep the program interesting as well.

FOLLOW THE BASICS

Initially, you will want to focus most of your energy on the diet and exercise instructions. These will provide you with the quickest, most visible results. The creative visualization exercises will also be beneficial, especially in maintaining motivation. In addition, choose one or two of the suggested techniques, such as the use of a dry skin brush, and perhaps schedule yourself for a weekly lymphatic massage or acupuncture session.

Supplements are not a requirement for your success on this program. While they can be beneficial, they are not a substitute for healthy diet and exercise habits.

ANTI-CELLULITE PROGRAM FLOW CHART

This flow chart is similar to the plan I follow. Yours should at least include the **bold-faced** suggestions. The other components are up to you. Just remember that the more you do to take care of yourself, the faster your Anti-Cellulite results will be. Study the flow chart and use it in conjunction with a journal to monitor yourself and chart your progress.

* Arise early enough to eat breakfast and exercise before leaving for work.
* Drink a small glass of fresh juice before exercise.
* **Follow your adaption of the Anti-Cellulite Exercise Program.**
* Dry Brush your skin.
* Shower, using a loofah to increase circulation.
* Apply nutrient-rich lotion to your skin after drying off.
* **Eat a breakfast of fresh fruit, or properly combined foods.**
* **Eat fresh vegetables plus a starch or protein for lunch.**
* Take five minutes of your lunch break to do a short Anti- Cellulite Visualization.

* Take a yoga class after work
* **Eat a dinner of vegetables with protein or starch**
* Listen to an Anti-Cellulite Visualization tape as you fall asleep.

If you do a few things during the day to treat yourself well and help your body, your body will take good care of you. There are so many benefits that come along by simply doing a few things to nurture yourself. Many of us are waiting for someone to take care of us. We are waiting for external forces (instead of internal ones) to compel us into self-care.

You are the only person responsible for yourself. If you wait for someone to fix you, you might never take charge of your life! It is so much easier to take **preventative** care, so that you don't have to wait for a disease to force you into change.

HABITS THAT AREN'T HELPING YOU

As you remember, the greatest contributing factor to your cellulite is toxins. Although you may not be able to entirely control environmental toxins, you are in control of what you put into your own body. You are the only one responsible for what you eat, drink or otherwise consciously consume. Each time you put something inside of your body you are making a choice *for* or *against* health.

Many people have at least one habit that is sabotaging their body in some way. Let's review some problem-causing habits and their possible relationship to the cellulite you're eliminating.

OVEREATING AND CELLULITE

Even the best of foods in excess can be detrimental to your health. You are the only one who can know how much is too much for you. Nowhere in this book is it written how much or how little you should eat. This is left completely up to you. If you feel you need advice concerning this, please consult your physician. Learn to feel how much your body is comfortable with. Eating slowly and consciously can help. Pay attention to how the food tastes, smells and feels in your mouth.

The reasons for overeating range from emotional needs to filling nutritional ones. You may be upset, angry or feel "empty", and fill the emotional black hole with too much food. This is no permanent solution. The only lasting results are fat and cellulite on the hips and thighs.

If emotional overeating is a problem, try to change the pattern by substituting another

activity. For example, instead of eating a piece
of cake when you're upset, you may want to
take a brisk walk around the block instead.
You will feel invigorated from your walk, instead
of guilty for eating the cake.

Your body may be hungry because of
incomplete absorbtion of nutrients. One cause
of this can be the result of years of accumulated
waste in the intestines. Nutrients are absorbed
in the small intestine. Tiny finger-like organs
called villi are responsible for this process.
When these villi become clogged and congested,
foods are not able to be metabolized and
utilized as efficiently as they should be. If the
small intestine is unable to absorb properly,
the body sends a message to the mind that it
needs more nourishment. Rather than crying
for more food, the body is actually crying for
more nutrients.

As you follow the Anti-Cellulite Diet
Program, you should find yourself gradually
losing the desire to overeat. The types of foods
you will be eating will not only promote the
cleansing of your intestines, but will be high in
nutrients as well.

ALCOHOLIC BEVERAGES
AND CELLULITE

Alcohol only adds to the toxins in your
body. Since you now know that toxins are a
direct cause of cellulite, it will be a conscious
act of creating more cellulite every time you

drink. If you do not want to give up alcohol, drink only moderately, for example on your "feast day".

Many women, especially in the premenstrual portion of their cycle, crave alcohol, claiming it helps them feel better. This may be related to blood sugar levels, which tend to be lower and less consistent at this time of the month. My mother discovered carrot juice cocktails as a substitution for alcoholic ones. This is a pleasant and effective alternative to alcohol. Not only is it non toxic, it is a wonderful stabilizer for low-blood sugar.

COFFEE AND CELLULITE

How many people do you know who *must* have their cup (or pot!) of coffee in the morning? This is the most common American habit, and is therefore not recognized for what it really is: an addiction.

Caffeine is a stimulant that directly affects the central nervous system. It has been linked to increased heart rate, irregular coronary circulation, increased blood pressure, birth defects, diabetes, and kidney failure. Coffee has been cited in several articles as a major contributing cause of cellulite.

Caffeine is not the only toxic substance in coffee. The coffee sold in the United States is primarily shipped to us from the Third World countries in which the coffee is grown.

There are in excess of ninety-four different pesticides used in Brazil, Columbia, Mexico and Guatemala. Only tiny samples are ever tested for illegal residues of pesticides, and often up to ten times the amount of chemicals legal in the U.S. are used in the growing process.

SMOKING AND CELLULITE

If you smoke, the smoke you're inhaling does not only affect your lungs. All bodily systems are interdependent. It is impossible to abuse only one part of the body and expect the other parts to look and feel normal. Smoking cigarettes is so poisonous that the Surgeon General's warning is required to be on cigarette package labels.

The cigarette habit is an addiction, and it is a very difficult one to break. Some people like to quit cold turkey, others prefer to wean themselves gradually. If you continue to smoke, your efforts to eliminate cellulite are sabotaged. You might consider joining a group program. Quitting smoking is another loving thing you can do for yourself and your body.

Because of the three-weeks-to-change-a-habit pattern you might consider quitting smoking before embarking on the Anti-Cellulite Program.

SUNTANNING AND CELLULITE

Excessive exposure to the sun causes skin damage. In addition, it has been shown that the collagen and elastin break down from long-term or high-intensity exposure to the sun's rays. As mentioned in Chapter 2, these are the very tissues which, when weakened, lead to an increase in cellulite.

Use a sun-protection cream or lotion while in the sun, especially during the hours from 10AM to 2PM. This will not only protect your skin, it will help prevent additional cellulite.

INACTIVITY AND CELLULITE

Disuse is self abuse. When you lead a sedentary life, your muscles, mind and being atrophy. You can help yourself change by imagining cellulite growing on your body with every couch-potato hour you sit in front of the television.

It's good to relax, and there's a difference between relaxing and being a couch potato. Why not use your break time to do some creative visualization techniques, take a walk, or go to the gym? You'll feel so much better afterwards.

GOOD HABITS
THAT WILL HELP YOU

The Anti-Cellulite Program has been designed to become a positive new lifestyle for you. It is not a crash program, and it is not depleting to your to system in any way. It is simply a collection of healthy habits to incorporate into your life. Many of these can take the place of some of the less healthy habits you may have had in the past.

When you feel healthy, it's much easier to live a happy and successful life. You've learned habits of exercise, diet, thinking and nurturing yourself. You've become familiar with elements of a healthy lifestyle that should become less and less of a program, and more and more of a way of life.

Chapter 9

THE ANTI-CELLULITE LIFE STYLE

You've arrived! In the past several chapters you have learned a lot about your body, your mind, and hopefully you have learned a little more about yourself. You have reviewed the causes of cellulite, and best of all you have discovered that there truly is a solution.

You no longer need to be resigned to having cellulite as the sign of an aging body. You merely need to recognize that when this orange peel appearance of the skin shows up on your body, it's an indication that your system needs some attention.

CELLULITE IS YOUR FRIEND

Cellulite has done you a favor. It has given you a signal that your body wants to be taken care of, and a reason to begin a healthier way of life. In fact, it will continue to do this for the rest of your life. It will appear only when your body needs it as a special messenger to call attention to your lifestyle and request a change.

ANTI-CELLULITE SUPPORT GROUPS

You might like to use this manual as a program guide to start an Anti-Cellulite support group. A support group can provide ongoing encouragement and the positive energy to keep you motivated. Now instead of complaining about cellulite, you can do something about it, *together!*

FITNESS TRAINERS

A personal fitness trainer can also be of help to you, especially during the first three weeks of the program. Meeting with a trainer at least once or twice a week is wonderful for those who could use the extra support and personal guidance. Make sure they have legitimate training, and don't be afraid to ask to see their certificate.

CONGRATULATIONS!
THE CELLULITE IS GONE!

Once your cellulite is gone, there is no need to be so strict with yourself in the areas of diet and exercise. Maintain all of the good habits you have acquired while on this program, but give yourself more leniency than while you were eliminating cellulite.

You should be forever free of cellulite if you follow the core Anti-Cellulite Program most of the time. Remember to have fun, and enjoy being fit, beautiful and alive. Wishing you continued health, self-love and success with your life!

With Love,

Laura Simms

Laura Simms

APPENDIX

I. TAKING YOUR PULSE

1. With the forefinger of one hand, find the pulsing artery on your opposite wrist, about one inch below the base of your thumb.
2. Count the number of beats in six seconds, using a wristwatch or a clock.
3. Multiply this number by ten (add zero to the number of heartbeats in six seconds) to obtain your current heart rate.

II. ESTABLISHING YOUR TARGET HEART RATE

1. Find your Resting Heart Rate (RHR) by taking your pulse for six seconds and multiplying by 10. It should be between 60-90. Take your pulse several times during the day, and determine your Resting Heart Rate by taking an average of five or six counts.
2. Then find your Maximum Heart Rate (MHR) by using the following formula.

Maximum Heart Rate = 220 minus your age
Example: 220-20= 200

147

3. Use Maximum Heart Rate (MHR) and your Resting Heart Rate (RHR) to find your Target Heart Rate (THR):

$$THR = .7(MHR-RHR) + RHR$$

For Example: .7(200-60) + 60
.7x140 + 60
98 + 60 = 158

THR=158

III. YOUR WORKOUT EQUIPMENT

If you do choose to work out at home, you will need to acquire the following equipment:

1. An exercise bench that can be adjusted to both flat and incline positions.
2. A bench press station to be fitted over your exercise bench.
3. A set of dumbbell weights, including two each of the following weights: five, eight, ten, twelve, fifteen, twenty, and twenty-five pounds.
4. A barbell set, including a twenty-pound bar with various poundages.
5. An exercise mat, approximately three by six feet, or more.
6. Ankle weights.

7. A full length mirror, to watch for correct exercise form.

It can be fairly expensive to set up your own home gym, but ultimately it is less costly than most gym memberships. You can purchase equipment through advertisers in fitness magazines like *Flex* and *Muscle and Fitness*, from the classified ads in your local newspaper or from a sporting goods store.

IV. RECOMMENDED READING LIST

DIET AND FOOD-COMBINING

Fit for Life
Harvey and Marilynn Diamond

Food Combining for Health
Doris Grant and Jean Joice

The McDougall Plan
John A McDougall, M.D. & Mary A. McDougall

WHOLISTIC HEALTH

The Holistic Health Lifebook
Bauman, E., Brint, A.I., Piper, L. and Wright, A.

Living Health
Harvey and Marilyn Diamond

Ayurveda:
     The Science of Self Healing
Dr. Vasant Lad

The McDougall Plan
John A McDougall, M.D. and
Mary A McDougall

VEGETARIAN COOKBOOKS

The New Laurel's Kitchen
Laurel Robertson

Enchanted Broccoli Forest
Mollie Katzen

The McDougall Health-Supporting Cookbook
Mary McDougall

EXERCISE

Now or Never
Joyce L. Vedral, Ph.D.

Perfect Parts
Rachel McLish

Fit or Fat
Covert Bailey

Stretching
Bob Anderson

CREATIVE VISUALIZATION
And Personal Growth

Creative Visualization
Shakti Gawain

You Can Heal Your Life
Louise Hay

Psycho-Cybernetics
Maltz, Maxwell, M.D.

Self Imagery: Creating Your Own Good Health
Emmet E. Miller, M.D.

V. THE CELLULITE SOLUTION PROGRESS LOG

The following seven pages include a progress log for you to chart your program on a daily basis. This will enable you to be aware of the changes your are making, and will also help in keeping you committed at the onset of the program.

If you feel you would like to chart more than one week, you have the author's permission to make copies of the chart for your own personal use. For best results, use this in conjunction with the Anti-Cellulite Flow Chart (p.135) and the Anti-Cellulite Goal Exercise (p.121).

THE CELLULITE SOLUTION PROGRESS LOG

Date: _____

— MONDAY —

	MORNING	AFTERNOON	EVENING
Anti-Cellulite **DIET**	Time: Item(s):	Time: Item(s):	Time: Item(s):
Anti-Cellulite **EXERCISE**	Time: Activities:	Time: Activities:	Time: Activities:
Anti-Cellulite **SUPPLEMENTS**	Time: Item(s):	Time: Item(s):	Time: Item(s):
Anti-Cellulite **WATER**	Time: # of 8oz. glasses:	Time: # of 8oz. glasses:	Time: # of 8oz. glasses:
Anti-Cellulite **TECHNIQUES**	Time: Technique:	Time: Technique:	Time: Technique:
Anti-Cellulite **MENTAL EXERCISES**	Time: Exercise:	Time: Exercise:	Time: Exercise:
Notes:			

THE CELLULITE SOLUTION PROGRESS LOG

Date: _____

— TUESDAY —

	MORNING	AFTERNOON	EVENING
Anti-Cellulite **DIET**	Time: Item(s):	Time: Item(s):	Time: Item(s):
Anti-Cellulite **EXERCISE**	Time: Activities:	Time: Activities:	Time: Activities:
Anti-Cellulite **SUPPLEMENTS**	Time: Item(s):	Time: Item(s):	Time: Item(s):
Anti-Cellulite **WATER**	Time: # of 8oz. glasses:	Time: # of 8oz. glasses:	Time: # of 8oz. glasses:
Anti-Cellulite **TECHNIQUES**	Time: Technique:	Time: Technique:	Time: Technique:
Anti-Cellulite **MENTAL EXERCISES**	Time: Exercise:	Time: Exercise:	Time: Exercise:
Notes:			

THE CELLULITE SOLUTION PROGRESS LOG

Date: _____

— WEDNESDAY —

	MORNING	AFTERNOON	EVENING
Anti-Cellulite **DIET**	Time: Item(s):	Time: Item(s):	Time: Item(s):
Anti-Cellulite **EXERCISE**	Time: Activities:	Time: Activities:	Time: Activities:
Anti-Cellulite **SUPPLEMENTS**	Time: Item(s):	Time: Item(s):	Time: Item(s):
Anti-Cellulite **WATER**	Time: # of 8oz. glasses:	Time: # of 8oz. glasses:	Time: # of 8oz. glasses:
Anti-Cellulite **TECHNIQUES**	Time: Technique:	Time: Technique:	Time: Technique:
Anti-Cellulite **MENTAL EXERCISES**	Time: Exercise:	Time: Exercise:	Time: Exercise:
Notes:			

THE CELLULITE SOLUTION PROGRESS LOG

Date: _____

— THURSDAY —

	MORNING	AFTERNOON	EVENING
Anti-Cellulite DIET	Time: Item(s):	Time: Item(s):	Time: Item(s):
Anti-Cellulite EXERCISE	Time: Activities:	Time: Activities:	Time: Activities:
Anti-Cellulite SUPPLEMENTS	Time: Item(s):	Time: Item(s):	Time: Item(s):
Anti-Cellulite WATER	Time: # of 8oz. glasses:	Time: # of 8oz. glasses:	Time: # of 8oz. glasses:
Anti-Cellulite TECHNIQUES	Time: Technique:	Time: Technique:	Time: Technique:
Anti-Cellulite MENTAL EXERCISES	Time: Exercise:	Time: Exercise:	Time: Exercise:
Notes:			

THE CELLULITE SOLUTION PROGRESS LOG

Date: _____

— FRIDAY —

	MORNING	AFTERNOON	EVENING
Anti-Cellulite **DIET**	Time: Item(s):	Time: Item(s):	Time: Item(s):
Anti-Cellulite **EXERCISE**	Time: Activities:	Time: Activities:	Time: Activities:
Anti-Cellulite **SUPPLEMENTS**	Time: Item(s):	Time: Item(s):	Time: Item(s):
Anti-Cellulite **WATER**	Time: # of 8oz. glasses:	Time: # of 8oz. glasses:	Time: # of 8oz. glasses:
Anti-Cellulite **TECHNIQUES**	Time: Technique:	Time: Technique:	Time: Technique:
Anti-Cellulite **MENTAL EXERCISES**	Time: Exercise:	Time: Exercise:	Time: Exercise:
Notes:			

THE CELLULITE SOLUTION PROGRESS LOG

Date: _____

— SATURDAY —

	MORNING	AFTERNOON	EVENING
Anti-Cellulite **DIET**	Time: Item(s):	Time: Item(s):	Time: Item(s):
Anti-Cellulite **EXERCISE**	Time: Activities:	Time: Activities:	Time: Activities:
Anti-Cellulite **SUPPLEMENTS**	Time: Item(s):	Time: Item(s):	Time: Item(s):
Anti-Cellulite **WATER**	Time: # of 8oz. glasses:	Time: # of 8oz. glasses:	Time: # of 8oz. glasses:
Anti-Cellulite **TECHNIQUES**	Time: Technique:	Time: Technique:	Time: Technique:
Anti-Cellulite **MENTAL EXERCISES**	Time: Exercise:	Time: Exercise:	Time: Exercise:
Notes:			

THE CELLULITE SOLUTION PROGRESS LOG

Date: _____

— SUNDAY —

	MORNING	AFTERNOON	EVENING
Anti-Cellulite **DIET**	Time: Item(s):	Time: Item(s):	Time: Item(s):
Anti-Cellulite **EXERCISE**	Time: Activities:	Time: Activities:	Time: Activities:
Anti-Cellulite **SUPPLEMENTS**	Time: Item(s):	Time: Item(s):	Time: Item(s):
Anti-Cellulite **WATER**	Time: # of 8oz. glasses:	Time: # of 8oz. glasses:	Time: # of 8oz. glasses:
Anti-Cellulite **TECHNIQUES**	Time: Technique:	Time: Technique:	Time: Technique:
Anti-Cellulite **MENTAL EXERCISES**	Time: Exercise:	Time: Exercise:	Time: Exercise:
Notes:			

VI. <u>FOOD COMBINING CHART</u>

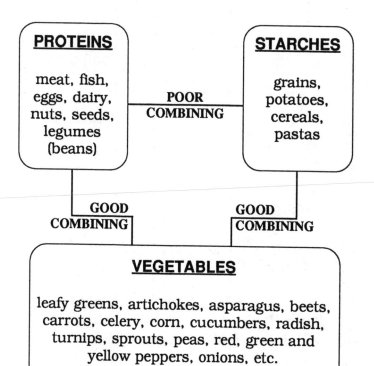

<u>PROTEINS</u>

meat, fish,
eggs, dairy,
nuts, seeds,
legumes
(beans)

**POOR
COMBINING**

<u>STARCHES</u>

grains,
potatoes,
cereals,
pastas

**GOOD
COMBINING**

**GOOD
COMBINING**

<u>VEGETABLES</u>

leafy greens, artichokes, asparagus, beets,
carrots, celery, corn, cucumbers, radish,
turnips, sprouts, peas, red, green and
yellow peppers, onions, etc.

Fruit should always be eaten alone

<u>FRUITS</u>

apples, apricots, bananas, grapes,
mangos, papayas, berries, oranges,
grapefruit, pineapple, etc.

BIBLIOGRAPHY

Books

Addington, Jack Ensign. All About Goals. Marina del Ray, CA: DeVorss & Company, 1977.

American Medical Association Book of Heartcare, New York, NY: Random House, 1982.

Anderson, Bob. Stretching. Bolinas, CA: Shelter Publishing., 1980.

Bailey, Covert. Fit or Fat? Boston, MA: Houghton Mifflin Co., 1978.

Bauman, E., Brint, A.I., Piper, L., Wright, A. The Holistic Health Lifebook. Berkeley, CA: Berkeley Holistic Health Center, 1981.

Carter, Albert E., The Miracles of Rebound Exercise. Edmonds, WA: The National Institute of Reboundology and Health, Inc., 1979.

Diamond, Harvey and Marilyn. Fit For Life. New York, NY: Warner Comm. Company, 1985.

Enzymatic Therapy, Formulas For Health, Health Guide No. 17: A Comprehensive Guide to Cellulite. Green Bay WI: Enzymatic Therapy, 1988.

160

Gawain, Shakti. Creative Visualization. San Rafael, CA: Whatever Publishing, Inc., 1978.

Gawain, Shakti. Living in the Light. San Rafael, CA: Whatever Publishing, Inc., 1986.

Grant, Doris and Joice, Jean. Food Combining for Health, Rochester, VT: Inner Traditions, 1987.

Hay, Louise, L. You Can Heal Your Life. Santa Monica, CA: Hay House, 1984.

Kirschmann, John D. Nutrition Almanac. New York, NY: McGraw-Hill Book Company, 1984.

Lad, Vasant. Ayurveda, The Science of Self-Healing. Santa Fe, NM: Lotus Press, 1985.

Lappe, Francis Moore. Diet for a Small Planet. Somersworth, NH, 1982.

Lark, Susan, M.D. Premenstrual Syndrome Self-Help Book. Los Angeles, CA: Forman Publishing, Inc.,1984.

Maltz, Maxwell, M.D. Psycho-Cybernetics. Hollywood, CA: Wilshire Book Co., 1960.

McDougall, John A., M.D. & Mary A. McDougall. The McDougall Plan. Piscataway, NJ: New Century Publishers, Inc., 1983.

McLish, Rachel. Perfect Parts. New York, NY: Warner Books, 1987.

Miller, Emmet, E. Self Imagery: Creating Your Own Good Health. Berkeley, CA: Celestial Arts, 1986.

Ray, Sondra. Celebration of Breath. Berkeley, CA: Celestial Arts, 1983.

Robbins, John. Diet for A New America, Walpole, NH: Stillpoint Publishing, 1987.

Roth, Geneen. Feeding the Hungry Heart. New York, NY: Signet, New American Library, 1982.

Rosnard, Nicole. Cellulite: Those lumps, bumps and bulges you couldn't lose before. New York, NY: Bantam Books, 1975.

Saifer, Phyllis, M.D., M.P.H., & Zellerbach, Merla. DETOX. New York, NY: Ballantine Books, 1984.

Van Gelder, Naneene, & Marks, Sheryl. Aerobic Dance-Exercise Instructor Manual. San Diego, CA: International Dance-Exercise Association (IDEA) Foundation, 1987.

Wesley-Hosford, Zia. The Beautiful Body Book. New York, NY: Bantam Books, 1989.

Yudkin, John. <u>The Penguin Encyclopaedia of Nutrition</u>. London, England: Penguin Books Ltd, 1985.

MAGAZINES

Glamour, Conde Nast Publications Inc. 350 Madison Ave, New York, NY, 10017.

Harper's Bazaar, The Hearst Corp. 1700 Broadway, New York, NY, 10019.

Muscle and Fitness, 21100 Erwin Street, Woodland Hills, CA 91367.

Prevention Magazine, Rodale Press, Inc. 33 E Minor St, Emmaus, PA, 18049.

Shape, 2110 Erwin Street, Woodland Hills, CA 92367.

Strength Training for Beauty, 1400 Stierlin Road, Mountain View, CA 94043

TAPES

DuBelle, Lee. <u>The Pre-Menstrual Syndrome Cellulite Connection</u>. Phoenix, Arizona, 1984

ABOUT THE AUTHOR

A native Californian, raised among the Redwoods in Eureka, Laura Simms became interested in health and nutrition under her family's influence. She attended Scripps College and graduated Phi Beta Kappa with a degree in music and a minor in humanities.

During college she began training with weights and continued to educate herself about nutrition and supplementation.

She currently lives in Southern California where she has received her Certification in Fitness Training from University of California, Irvine. Through her work at a natural grocery store, Laura continues to keep abreast of the latest developments in vitamins, supplements and natural cosmetics. In addition she is a personal fitness trainer, maintaining as many clients as time will allow.

INDEX

Acidophilus, 98
Acupressure, 82
Acupuncture, 81
Addictive substances, 43
Additives, 42-43
Aerobic, defined, 62
Affirmations, 127-129
Alcoholic Beverages, 138-139
Aloe Vera, 98
Amino acids, 94-96, 108-109
Anderson, Bob, 150
Anti-Cellulite
  benefits of visualization, 115
  diet, purpose of, 31
  exercise program, 2, 22, 57-75
  food combining, 44, 159
  mind power exercises, 119
Anti-Oxidant nutrients, 102
Artificial sweeteners, 42
Asanas, 83

Bailey, Covert, 150
Bauman, E., 149
Beans, 35
Bee pollen, 98
Beta carotene, 99
Bio flavinoids, 99
Bladderwrack, 93
Blood, 18, 24
Body wraps, herbal, 105

Gotu Kola, 92
Grains, 34
Grant, Doris, 149
Guar Gum, 99

Hay Louise, 117-118, 151
Heart rate, 147-148
Herbal body wraps, 105
Herbs, 88, 92-93
Holistic, x
Hormones, 16, 18
Hypertension, 25
Hypoglycemia, 16

Immune system, 20
Inactivity, 141
Injury guidelines, 75
Inosine, 199
Inositol, 97

Juices, 37
Joice, Jean, 149

Katzen, Mollie, 150

L-Carnitine, 94-95
L-Cysteine, 95
L-Methionine, 95
L-Taurine, 96
L-Threonine, 95
Lad, Dr. Vasant, 150
Legumes, 35

lipotropic, 101-102
minerals, 97-98
question and answers on, 105-109
superfoods, 98-100
vitamins, 96-97
Support groups, 144

Testosterone, 60
Thoracic duct, 19
Tissue, 13, 14

Vedral, Ph.D., Joyce L., 150
Vegetables, 33
Visualization, 112-116, 123-125, 129-131
Vitamins, 96-97

Warm up, 69
Water, 37, 89-91
Water retention, 17
Wheat bread substitutes, 34
Wheat four products, 38-39
White flour products, 38-39
Whole body lymphatic massage, 81
Wholistic, x
Wright, A., 149

Yoga, 65, 82

Zinc, 98

The Cellulite Solution

Self Care Products Personally Selected by Laura:

Mineral Bath Salts, 9 oz. $7.95
Skin Brush, with detachable handle 7.95
Loofah, one medium size 2.95
The Cellulite Solution Visualization Tape........9.95
       Side 1: Visualization
       Side 2: Positive Affirmations

'The Kit' 24.95
       includes all of the above (Save 3.85!)

The Cellulite Solution, book:
       one copy .... 12.95 ea.
       two or three copies .... 10.95 ea.
       four or five copies ....9.50 ea.
       six or more - ....Call for price

The Cellulite Newsletter. Current information,
tips to success, evaluation of new products and
techniques, etc. Six issue per year.
Written by Laura Simms 15.00/year

Twenty-One Day Menu Planner. Compliments and
extends information provided in the book. Includes
many delicious and healthful recipies.
Written by Laura Simms 7.95

Toll Free # 800-333-4593

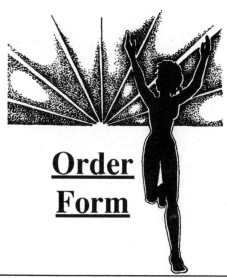

Order Form

Quantity	Product Ordered	Price	Total
	Subtotal		
	CA residents add 7.75% state sales tax		
	Shipping & Handling		3.50
	Total		

To order, call toll-free 800-333-4593,

or send check or money order to:
Infonex Corp.
1130 Calle Cordillera, Suite 102
San Clemente, Ca. 92672

Visa or MasterCard # _____ Exp. Date: _____

Signature: _____

If you are not <u>completely</u> satisfied with anything you purchase your money will be promptly and pleasantly refunded.